"I think the book is an important, creative, thoughtful contribution to gestalt therapy research and practice. It is suitable for both those interested in research, and those interested in deepening their clinical sensibilities. Adam's ability to intermingle history/culture/politics with specific moments-in-living is rare. But once you lean into it, I think one never hears clinical material (or their own stories) in quite the same way again. He expands our boundaries of inclusiveness."

Lynne Jacobs, PhD, Co-founder of Pacific Gestalt Institute;
Training and Supervising Analyst, Institute of
Contemporary Psychoanalysis

"No excuses! Pay attention right there where you turn your sight away – both outwards and inwards. This is how this work builds painful sensitivity to minorities of all kinds – both outwards and inwards. All this done with a systematic curiosity (this is research) and touching boldness (it is just Adam). We see autoethnography bridging research with life: we want to read more about Adam because we want to know more about ourselves."

Jan Roubal, MD, PhD, Masaryk University
in Brno, Czech Republic; gestalt therapy
trainer and supervisor

"The use of autoethnography to explore, interrogate, and challenge aspects of therapy culture is always welcome. Adam does this in fascinating, courageous, and engaging ways in this text. His work exemplifies high quality research which unashamedly celebrates subjectivity in therapy-focused autoethnographic inquiry. In a study that gets close into the interconnection of the personal with the cultural in gestalt therapy, he does a great service to that modality. Arcane sacred cows always need to be scrutinised, challenged, and Adam certainly does this in ways that are scholarly, insightful, and fun. The gestalt community should rejoice!"

Alec Grant, PhD, independent scholar; co-editor of
Contemporary British Autoethnography and
*International Perspectives on Autoethnographic
Research and Practice*

"You have in front of you a landmark book that deserves attention on many different counts. Readers of *Exploring Masculinity, Sexuality, and Culture in Gestalt Therapy: An Autoethnography* will be rewarded with a stimulating variety of challenging topics – some of them familiar in today's field-relational gestalt discourse, and others which break new ground, practically and conceptually. Throughout the book, the author's purposefulness and professionalism are displayed in full, as well as his ethical priorities, his openness to LGBTQ perspectives, his courage in displaying so much of his personal truth, and a lot more."

From the Foreword by Malcolm Parlett,
PhD, the author of *Future Sense*

W0234923

Exploring Masculinity, Sexuality, and Culture in Gestalt Therapy

Exploring Masculinity, Sexuality, and Culture in Gestalt Therapy is an invitation to explore social and political issues within the psychotherapeutic framework. It describes and analyses the author's journey of becoming a gestalt therapist in Poland and England through analyses of masculinity, sexuality, relationality, and culture.

This book addresses the collective gestalts exploring the psychotherapeutic taboos of sexual transference, same-sex attraction, use or lack of touch, gender equality, and inter-cultural conflicts. Each chapter is an exploration of prejudices embedded in our cultures and therapeutic work, and provides a theoretical challenge to current practices within gestalt therapy and beyond. The author advocates for a more collective understanding of embodied sensations emerging in the therapeutic context as collective gestalts.

Through the use of autoethnographic research methodology, this book shows how personal embodied experiences are intertwined with the social, political, and material context. It is essential reading for gestalt therapists, as well as readers interested in gestalt approaches.

Adam Kincel is a gestalt therapist, supervisor, and trainer based in the UK. His work focuses on the co-emergence of embodied relational therapy and political issues.

The Gestalt Therapy Book Series

Scientific Board

The Istituto di Gestalt series of gestalt therapy books emerges from the ground of a growing interest in theory, research and clinical practice in the Gestalt community. The members of the Scientific and Editorial Boards have been committed for many years to the process of supporting research and publications in our field: through this series we want to offer our colleagues internationally the richness of the current trends in Gestalt therapy theory and practice, underpinned by research. The goal of this series is to develop the original principles in hermeneutic terms: to articulate a relational perspective, namely a phenomenological, aesthetic, field-oriented approach to psychotherapy. It is also intended to help professions and to support a solid development and dialogue of gestalt therapy with other psychotherapeutic methods.

The series includes original books specifically created for it, as well as translations of volumes originally published in other languages. We hope that our editorial effort will support the growth of the gestalt therapy community; a dialogue with other modalities and disciplines; and new developments in research, clinics and other fields where gestalt therapy theory can be applied (e.g., organizations, education, political and social critique and movements).

We would like to dedicate this Gestalt Therapy Book Series to all our masters and colleagues who have sown fruitful seeds in our minds and hearts.

Human interaction and Emotional Awareness in Gestalt Therapy
Exploring the Phenomenology of Contacting and Feeling
Peter H. Dreitzel

For more information on the titles in this series, please visit www.routledge.com/ Gestalt-Therapy/book-series/GESTHE and www.gestaltitaly.com

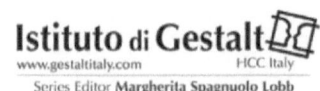

Istituto di Gestalt
www.gestaltitaly.com   HCC Italy
Series Editor **Margherita Spagnuolo Lobb**

Exploring Masculinity, Sexuality, and Culture in Gestalt Therapy

An Autoethnography

Adam Kincel

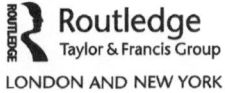

Routledge
Taylor & Francis Group

LONDON AND NEW YORK

First published 2021
by Routledge
2 Park Square, Milton Park, Abingdon, Oxon OX14 4RN

and by Routledge
52 Vanderbilt Avenue, New York, NY 10017

Routledge is an imprint of the Taylor & Francis Group, an informa business

British Library Cataloguing-in-Publication Data
A catalogue record for this book is available from the British Library

Library of Congress Cataloging-in-Publication Data
Names: Kincel, Adam, author.
Title: Exploring masculinity, sexuality, and culture in gestalt
   therapy : an autoethnographic / Adam Kincel.
Description: Milton Park, Abingdon, Oxon ; New York, NY :
   Routledge, 2021. | Series: Gestalt therapy books series |
   Includes bibliographical references and index.
Identifiers: LCCN 2020034330 (print) | LCCN 2020034331 (ebook) |
   ISBN 9780367633059 (hardback) | ISBN 9780367633066 (paperback) |
   ISBN 9781003118732 (ebook)
Subjects: LCSH: Gestalt therapy. | Psychotherapy. | Ethnology.
Classification: LCC RC489.G4 K56 2021 (print) | LCC RC489.G4 (ebook) |
   DDC 616.89/143—dc23
LC record available at https://lccn.loc.gov/2020034330
LC ebook record available at https://lccn.loc.gov/2020034331

ISBN: 978-0-367-63305-9 (hbk)
ISBN: 978-0-367-63306-6 (pbk)
ISBN: 978-1-003-11873-2 (ebk)

Typeset in Times New Roman
by Apex CoVantage, LLC

Contents

Figures

Tables

Foreword by Malcolm Parlett

You have in front of you a landmark book that deserves attention on many different counts. Readers of *Exploring Masculinity, Sexuality, and Culture in Gestalt Therapy: An Autoethnography* will be rewarded with a stimulating variety of challenging topics – some of them familiar in today's field-relational gestalt discourse, and others which break new ground, practically and conceptually. Throughout the book, the author's purposefulness and professionalism are displayed in full, as well as his ethical priorities, his openness to LGBTQ perspectives, his courage in displaying so much of his personal truth, and a lot more.

Adam Kincel writes from the perspective of an experienced gestalt psychotherapist and international trainer who is looking back on his personal and professional life from its very beginning. In effect, the book is an extended case study compiled by the author, in which – unusually – the subject of the study is the author himself. He researches and documents major events and themes that have arisen in his life, and reflects on what he discovers, recalls, and has over time worked through in therapy or has written up as part of his research journal – a feature of the methodology he adopts. He also interviews key family members (the interviews were significant events in themselves), and has focused conversations with therapist colleagues.

Advancing knowledge of self, being aware of present experience, and becoming "aware of one's awareness process", are vital elements in the serious practice of gestalt therapy and in the development of an overall "phenomenological attitude" (Yontef, 1993). Adam Kincel takes this important function to a whole new level. He accomplishes this by utilising a sophisticated research methodology – "autoethnography" – to investigate his life and development. Though others have written about their experience of receiving gestalt therapy, as far as I know this mode of inquiry has not been formally applied before in gestalt therapy. In this way, as in many others, *Exploring Masculinity, Sexuality, and Culture in Gestalt Therapy* breaks new ground.

There is strong philosophical underpinning for what he does and how he goes about it. There's very different epistemology in the choice of method used. *Ethnography* is the study and systematic recording of human cultures; *autoethnography* is the pursuit of such study by documenting the researcher's experience of living within – and being impacted by – his or her own culture. The narrative here pivots around Adam's passage from child to adult, and from boyhood interests in Poland all the way to his work as a present-day gestalt practitioner in Britain. His parents and home life obviously feature, but also education and friendships, difficulties and achievements, fantasies and shaming moments, and a whole range of adolescent challenges and choice points are explored in this account. But his experiences never appear in psychological isolation: they are observed in the lived-in contexts of family, society, culture, nationality; and in conjunction with prevalent ideologies, powerful historical and economic forces, and embedded networks of assumptions and expectations (e.g. about gender, class differences, and purposes of education) as they existed during the time and location of his growing up.

As the book's choice of title indicates, Adam concentrates on highly charged themes in his developmental journey, namely his growing sexual interests and attractions, his body changes in puberty and emergence of his masculine identity, and how he explored – and sometimes didn't allow himself to express – particular feminine as well as masculine qualities. This is an account of his immersion in the immediate milieu in which he grew, and the struggles he endured to find and live his truth. Clarifying his sexual identity involved creative adjustment and experimenting within the framework of pervasive norms, expectations, and pressures to conform that surrounded him.

The case study moves from his experiences as a sensitive boy emotionally overwhelmed by his overly affectionate mother, through the trials he faced on a "rough" working-class estate where he was perceived to be middle-class and "different", and how he hid in a concrete stairwell, was bullied, and survived this period through distracting himself – for a long stretch by playing computer games. He was already computer-addicted as a young boy – an ongoing source of parental concern.

His account is startlingly bold. We are admitted to aspects of personal life that most of us would probably not want to mention, let alone describe in detail. Adam, by contrast, records his life and conditions as he experienced them; the hazards and dangers he faced or resourcefully avoided; the disappointments and his times of feeling shame and deficiency; and a selection of quiet triumphs and happy successes (like his first kiss). Readers who do not already know Adam Kincel, and "meet" him here for the first time, are likely to be astonished at times at how open, frank, and undefended he is; readers who know him already will not be surprised: the same straightforward and open contact style which is evident in meeting him is evident in the book.

At points when some of us writing about our lives might be tempted to decorate or underline our achievements and breakthroughs, Adam consistently downplays them. A significant moment that stands out for me was when he comes to recognise the severity of his addiction to his computer. What does he do? He decides to sell it, which he sets about doing immediately, and discards a major support in his life. This entails a complete re-orientation of his non-school life. His parents cannot believe it, and are enthralled at the change. But this clearly is not an action taken to get his parents off his back; it's obvious to the reader that it's a moment of chosen release from a form of bondage: it is an act of agency that self-cures, and represents another step on the path to his maturity.

The practice of autoethnography entails Adam Kincel being both research investigator and meaning-maker-in-chief: he is the final arbiter of what to include and exclude. The methodological discipline has its own checks and obligations, but none of it is heavily prescriptive. There is not an exact rubric, but rather an invitation to construct an intelligent, flexible, and individually crafted research design process. For example, when he conducts interviews – for instance with his mother and his sister – there are expectations that certain procedures and safeguards need to be built-in, and he agonises over the ethics. Choosing how to conduct the meetings, and arranging, recording, and analysing the interviews become parts of the methodology he adopts.

I am underlining the methodology because, as a fellow member of the gestalt community, I am grateful to Adam Kincel for pioneering an exciting branch of research that deserves serious note. He is extending the range of possible approaches for other investigators to draw upon. He sets an example to follow and establishes a precedent of high standards. The approach is "gestalt friendly" in that it does justice to the complexity, multidimensionality, and honouring of subjectivity that accompany any profound investigation of an actual human life. As a form of phenomenological inquiry it permits and enables the researcher to alight on significant life themes without apology.

Gone are the known traps that many researchers fall into – parading so-called "objectivity" that denies the inherent subjectivity that lurks behind the front; crunching numbers to extract a trickle of human significance; and undue hesitancy around topics through fear of academic disapproval. That he ties his work together with some of the most radical contemporary research thinking in the social sciences has the effect of building a bridge to, and from, the gestalt therapy tradition. It is a bridge that I hope will carry a lot more traffic.

Another strength of the book is that Adam Kincel – supported by autoethnography – travels deeply into territory that belongs within the gestalt perimeter, but often has not been explored as comprehensively as it deserves. Let me explain the connections to field theory and Paul Goodman.

Central to a developed gestalt understanding is to recognise how many of the divisions in our society's general thinking are unhelpful, to say the least. Examples are well-known: splitting thought from feeling, or rational argument from emotional investment, need regular challenging. They represent the tendency to compartmentalise, which fails to match holistic phenomena as actually experienced. Splits of these kinds can even at times be fixed in concrete, with different university departments in separate buildings upholding and protecting their "specialities". Sometimes a new discipline can squeeze in to fill an obvious gap, rather as social psychology originally grew in the once unoccupied space between sociology and psychology; but the overwhelming tendency is to continue working within the confines of a single framework, thus reinforcing the fault lines of conventional thinking without challenging them.

What Adam Kincel does here is to show how crucial dimensions of human development have to be understood NOT as constituting a free-standing psychophysical progression, that is admittedly affected somewhat by "the environment", but as something far greater and more interesting. What his developed scrutiny reveals is an unfolding expression of the complete indivisibility of what was happening to him as "body" and what was happening to him as "cultural participant". He shows these cannot be discussed separately: they necessarily are to be known together. His vision opens out from the intimate realm of his boyhood life – including the physiological changes, and first attractions – to unpick the powerful cultural framework that operated in Poland about to emerge from under Soviet rule in the time of his growing up, and which formed an inescapable totality that he experienced, and which he experienced viscerally.

Gestalt has been here before. Adam Kincel is a worthy descendant of Paul Goodman in that he spans individual and society in a single inclusive sweep of his attention. To go back to basics, one of the most significant phrases in Perls, Hefferline, and Goodman (1951) is the "organism-environment field" with the crucial linking hyphen: the introduction of the term "field" bringing a person and their context together, regarding them as so intimately interwoven that they call for a single, or "unitary" approach to investigate them. There is no such thing as a contextless person, and no such thing as a context that is not suffused with personal input, imprint, and presence. Underlying Goodman's vision is what is addressed again in this book: the fundamental unity, and the erasure of the common dualism, between culture and body. Here is a re-statement and a welcome reminder of a central gestalt truth.

However, I suggest the argument here is more than a re-statement – that Kincel takes a further step. Within gestalt therapy thought and practice, the two constituents of the field rarely receive equal attention: usually the organism wins convincingly over the environment; we make the latter "ground": we attend to the personal story more than to the social, political, and cultural context in which the story unfolds. The very phrase "*organism-environment field*" almost establishes what's considered primary; and perhaps sometimes we need to reverse the order and think about the "*environment-organism field*" in order to correct the imbalance. This is what Adam strives to achieve, giving the full weight due to the background conditions in his family life, the urban housing estate they lived in, and the state institutions and economic conditions that existed in Poland during the years of his growing up and through the formative stages of his sexual developmental journey. Of many well-chosen quotations in Adam's book, one in particular stood out for me: Gadamer's remarks (in Section 2.3) that, "In fact history does not belong to us; we belong to it", and, "The self-awareness of the individual is only a flickering in the closed circuits of historical life". This insight captures exactly the need for the kind of re-balancing which is displayed so convincingly in this book.

There's another way to appreciate *Exploring Sexuality, Masculinity, and Culture* that is important to note. Adam Kincel is investigating his life. His work is an odyssey in what I call "self-recognising" (Parlett, 2015). In self-recognising we assimilate life's experience over time, acquire or search for memories, have new insights, discern patterns and life themes spread over years, and take ever wider existential perspectives that many (though not all) define as spiritual. I think of self-recognising as being a critical ingredient in what people think of as developing wisdom. Adam is doing something in a particular, systematic way that probably a majority of people do unsystematically at certain points in their life, for instance after a relational break-up or as they approach their death: they look back, remember, create or adjust their life narrative, review what they did or didn't do – maybe as a prelude to changing direction.

Arguably, the greatest gestalt contribution to psychotherapy is our emphasis on the here-and-now, and our attention to what is alive and present in the consulting room. There may therefore be hesitancy in endorsing activities that seem to centre on unearthing the past, or require "talking about" rather than direct and immediate experience. If this is a remaining traditional stance, it is good that this book may unsettle it. Adam shows clearly how making sense of his cumulative lived experience is healthy and necessary as part of his development and liberation. We all need to self-recognise – discover, for instance, those deeply habitual patterns that Fritz Perls labelled "character" that others can see more clearly than we can ourselves; and take the courageous and difficult subsequent steps, such as hearing others' feedback about our shortcomings and "blind spots", or unearth archaic events and traumatic episodes that we have avoided as too troubling to address. Self-recognising is not for wimps.

I have suggested that Adam Kincel has a strong connection to Paul Goodman. More surprisingly, perhaps, is a way that he follows Fritz Perls who, in his account of his life, his beliefs, and his ongoing existential themes, also engaged in self-recognising, even if he did not call it that. In my view, his book, *In and Out the Garbage Pail* (1969), has been underrated. The fact that it appeared at first without page numbers and with Russ Youngreen's playful drawings was all part of Perls himself making light of it, deflecting from what in fact it was – an intimate reflection on his life, a re-visiting of the past, a speculative analysis of how he had become who he was in the light of multiple influences (his parents, two world wars, his troubles with Freud, his relations with Lore), and his journey to gestalt pre-eminence. Perls moves between reminiscence and remembering – excavating the past – and his (then) present life at Esalen, including his ups and downs in the writing itself, as he freely imports countless anecdotes, snatches of poetry, and some newly generated thoughts.

In style and orderliness, Perls's slapdash-seeming account is as far away from Adam's ordered autoethnography as one could imagine. But there are fundamental similarities as well. Each of them is passionate and self-revealing; each uncovers the past as if to know it for the first time. Both acknowledge seriously difficult times, yet both have resilient confidence that the direction of life is sound and living to the full is ultimately the path. And central to both is the continual back-and-forth traffic between the past and the present – what happened for each of them *then*, and how it appears *now*, affirming that this is always the path to healing and integration (then and now!). Pointing to similarities should not mean ignoring some essential differences, of course. Writing in different eras, Adam's sensitivity to matters of gender, abuse, and the ethics of protection is totally different from that of his predecessor.

When it comes to knowing how much gestalt practitioners engage in self-recognising, when their initial training is over, there is only hearsay. While some of us continue to dig away at recalcitrant life patterns and self-destructive behaviour that we recognise, and may seek therapeutic help to contain or dismantle, there may be others who have long given up the habit of self-research, believing their long-ago personal development experiences and therapy at the time of training were sufficient for their lifetime (hopefully, others around them would agree). Potentially, what autoethnography provides is another form of inquiry, different from therapy but no less demanding, and maybe worth the effort. I think a case could be made that systematic unpicking of one's early life – as demonstrated here by Adam Kincel – while not being therapy as such, still constitutes a powerful discovery process from which many could benefit.

In my own self-work, for instance, historical research into British life during the war, especially 1940–42, has widened my vision and helped me integrate my early life experiences. But such research was never suggested in the course of extensive therapy. Now, with my (coaching) clients, when they connect present difficulties to earlier eras, I realise I am more inquisitive regarding physical, social, and economic conditions that framed the milieu in which they were living or working at the time, and I encourage their own research – which they take to enthusiastically. For those in the gestalt community, a wider application of auto-ethnography principles – looking back in time – may appear too near to the psychoanalytic tradition to be comfortable. But that misses the point that our social, political, and personal histories are inseparable aspects of our ground, shaping our present experience ineradicably. So my personal hope would be that collectively we might encourage self-research on autoethnographic lines as a supplementary framework for exploring how we developed as we did – again, putting "the environment" nearer to the centre of our awareness than therapists have been used to doing systematically.

An objection may be made that autoethnography and similar self-recognising pursuits are narcissistic. This is very superficial. In some circles, psychotherapy itself can be labelled "solipsistic and self-absorbed". Self-directed investigations of one's own life in depth and detail may seem to go even further in this direction. However, narcissism, marked by self-importance and need for attention and admiration, is exactly the kind of delusion and hidden fearfulness that could not survive a critical investigation of self of the kind that autoethnography requires. Adam has written (in a personal communication), that "autoethnography when properly done is about being vulnerable and showing all parts of ourselves" . . . the criteria are about "authenticity, multidimensionality". And if improperly done, what then? His reply was as follows: "The criteria to distinguish between good and bad autoethnography are aesthetic – an autoethnography of someone who is un-aware of their narcissistic wound would be rather boring. They would be defended, rigid and manipulative". As the book convincingly shows, Adam Kincel is not remotely any of these – indeed, he's almost the polar opposite. And the book is never boring.

The more general point is that in self-recognising there is always the potentiality for any of us to be unaware of certain qualities or habitual patterns of responding to our situations; but that does not invalidate the activity of self-recognising: rather it calls for *more* of it, with more rigour, depth, courage to question, and to get others' feedback, so that we can become aware of our previous unawareness.

I began this foreword by saying this is a landmark book. I hope I have shown you why I consider it a notable addition to the gestalt literature. The book deserves – and will receive – close study, for it opens doors that readers will want to open and find out more: it's that kind of book.

I am aware of two points that I have not made but I will sneak in at the end.

First, this book is especially thought-provoking for anyone who works as a body-psychotherapist. Much of Adam Kincel's journey in therapy was body-oriented, and some was helpful and some decidedly not. As part of the body emphasis, there is also a wise contribution to the debate around "touching clients".

Second, this is undoubtedly a book of importance for the LGBTQ community – Adam experienced homophobia at a cultural level in Poland at that point when he was unclear about his sexual identity. The account here engages with heteronormativity, gender stereotypes, and – again – readers will appreciate his wise and full contribution, his sympathetic treatment, and generous self-disclosure. As elsewhere, his knowledge of the specialist literature(s) will make this an indispensable book to return to, for many years to come.

It is the time for me to release your attention and hand over to Adam Kincel. I believe that he has done an excellent job in reporting his innovative research in stimulating fashion, revealing to a wide audience a distinctive form of investigation, with huge potential for future directions in gestalt therapy and beyond. I regard his work as a contemporary achievement of the first order, and my expectation is that at the end, readers will have a similar sense to my own – that of feeling privileged to have read it.

References

Parlett, M. (2015) *Future Sense: Five Explorations of Whole Intelligence for a World That's Waking Up.* Leicester: Troubador.

Perls, F.S. (1969) *In and Out the Garbage Pail.* Lafayette, CA: Real People Press.

Perls, F.S., Hefferline, R. and Goodman, P. (1951/1994) *Gestalt Therapy, Excitement and Growth in the Human Personality.* New York: Gestalt Journal Press.

Yontef, G.M. (1993) *Awareness, Dialogue and Process: Essays on Gestalt Therapy.* Highland, NY: Gestalt Journal Publications.

Acknowledgements

The completion of any work is a synergetic fusion of one's creativity and the support within one's environment. There are a huge number of people who supported me on my journey and here I would like to thank some of them.

Drs Alec Grant, Laetitia Zeeman, and Nichola Khan for holding me emotionally and intellectually through regular academic supervision, and their diligence and suggestion to explore post-structuralism and new materialism. All participants in this research that cannot be named for ethical reasons but who have had a significant impact on my life, career and this book. Toni Gilligan for the academic advice, trusting my clinical skills and inspiring me to develop and attend to my social self. Dr Lynne Jacobs for her supportive critique, enthusiasm about the issues that I consider in this book, and threatening me when I considered withdrawing from my psychotherapy training. Drs Katy Wakelin and Malcolm Parlett for editing my almost final work and intellectually stimulating, heart-opening hikes. Jen Leong for scribbling on the margins of my draft. Carol Siederer for her eyes lighting each time I asked her to discuss my doctorate in my clinical supervision. Piotr Mierkowski for reading my drafts and not retroflecting (holding back) when appraising and criticising. The remaining members of the British Gestalt Journal Writers Group that have not been included earlier: Dr Belinda Harris, Dr Christine Stevens, Jacqui Lichtenstern, John Gillespie, Lynne Brighouse, Martin Capps and Vivienne Barnett for providing physical and emotional space for my personal writing; Hannah Standen for being patient when correcting my written English and for her belief that I have the skills that doctoral training requires; Anna Taterka for the collaboration that led to the creation of the book cover and drawings presented in this study; Kasia Zając for her ongoing support and commitment to my various life projects; Michelle Billies for sharing her knowledge and expertise; as well as Jane Pennington for the final proofreading.

It is also important to acknowledge the supportive conditions of Tŷ Newydd, the National Writing Centre of Wales, and the experimental township of Auroville where most of this book was written.

Chapter 1

Welcome

I am struggling to write today. The book is almost completed, but the introduction is proving to be the most difficult part. I spent the whole day checking my emails and convincing myself that I have more urgent things to do. I don't stick to the plan that I created for this very luxurious week that I reserved for writing, but my feelings are shouting that I am not ready. I am not ready to become an author. I am afraid of exposing myself, of the reactions or perhaps rejection of the text as it talks about sexuality and cultural prejudices, and at the end, who am I to publish a book?

Would notes like that have any value for research and gestalt writing? We all make these notes. Sometimes they are mental notes, while sometimes we may even write them down. More often, we would discuss similar feelings with our friends or support groups, but can we use them in research that can contribute to current knowledge and develop gestalt therapy? Before I attempt to answer this question, let us explore what this text can offer. It is undoubtedly an intimate text, a disclosure that is often shared with people who are close by. Autobiographical writing brings about an intimacy that is hard to obtain in more recognisable research studies that use questionnaires or a series of interviews. This text shows specific issues that are relevant to me but can also be applicable to some readers: the struggle to find time for writing, fears of exposure and shame when exploring sexuality, a critical, shaming voice when exercising creativity, and integrating the new identity of an author. My assumption is that I am not writing only about myself, but that readers may identify with some of these themes. The method that I applied to my research and want to promote in this book is called autoethnography. It provides a method of analysing personal reflection from the perspectives of individuals embedded in them. In gestalt language, autoethnography looks for the background that created the figure, and the figure is the author's own becoming. Writing the text changes the author and, in this exercise, a new identity is created; this is why I always see it as becoming rather than who has become.

This book started as an experiment of embodiment that gave no guarantees. By attending to my body, the body of a gestalt therapist, various feelings, thoughts, contexts, and theories were born and recorded. Chapter after chapter, the focus and pattern started to emerge which eventually created a critique of the embodiment of culture, sexuality, and masculinity within gestalt therapy. As we are always embedded within a culture, this book suggests a revision of how therapists engage with clients from an inescapably prejudiced place. It is an invitation to therapists to deconstruct the "safe therapy" (Samuels, 2003) that avoids difficult subjects such as sexuality, gender, and culture by providing examples of the therapist's prejudices, heteronormativity, and hegemonic (the rigid, strong, sexually assertive, and dominating) masculinity from the therapy room to the researcher's private life. All theory is illustrated by personal examples, family photographs, and drawings to show the inseparability of the private and the cultural.

The purpose of this book can be encapsulated in three aims. The first one is to broaden the understanding of the relationship between body and culture within gestalt therapy. It is important for me, however, that this knowledge is not only theoretical but also able to be applied practically. Hence the second aim is to provide several examples of how to work practically with what is cultural in the intimacy of one-to-one therapy or larger group settings. The third aim is to familiarise gestalt therapists with autoethnographic research methodology that fits with gestalt therapy philosophies, while allowing us to find yet another way of communicating the beauty of our work to a wider group of researchers.

This book explores my embodied experience as inescapably cultural. Although gestalt therapy uses phenomenology to study embodied sensations, the focus here is on embodied sensations as a way to gain an understanding of our emotions in relation to the other. The work presented in this study extends the usual understanding of phenomenology in gestalt therapy, discussing how embodied sensations, breathing patterns, body posture, sense of space, awareness or lack of awareness of sensations, and other embodiments are dependent on collective political and social circumstances.

Furthermore, the embodiment of collective experiences is not presented only as a theoretical construct; this study also concerns the practicalities of attending to collective situations in the consulting room, psychotherapy training, and even the psychotherapist's private life: how therapists can zoom in and out to see the interplay between the current relational aspects and the wider socio-political situation. Through various examples, this research study examines the opportunities for dialogue, be it a large group, an intimate psychotherapy session, a training group, or personal relationship that build the necessary safety and trust to discuss but not avoid our prejudice. The concept of safe emergency (Perls, Hefferline and Goodman, 2003, pp. 277–289; Swanson, 1982) is central to the argument and means a way of creating safe conditions for attending to the uncomfortable political struggles that emerge as phenomenological sensations within current psychotherapeutic situations. As embodied cognition starts with the sensation, the body is for embodied research and the psychotherapist as a microscope is for the microbiologist.

Research methodologies are languages in which various tribes of researchers can understand each other. Autoethnography is not only a language that gestalt therapists can easily learn but also a language that has some words and grammar structure that we may want to adopt. This research methodology sees the individual as always embedded in the field of relationships and aims at deconstructing, unsettling the "I". Although talking about oneself may seem narcissistic, autoethnography invites us to show vulnerability, an authentic way of relating, to critique oneself and be open for other people's critique – actions that will scare people who are invested in maintaining a fixed image of themselves.

In the remaining part of the opening chapter, I am going to briefly introduce those readers who have not studied gestalt therapy to this modality, introduce autoethnography, which will be further discussed in Chapter 7, say a few words about my family who consented to this research study, and provide an overall structure and guidance about this book and how to read it.

1.1 Case study as an introduction to gestalt therapy

As an introduction to gestalt therapy and my work, I will present a short case study from training that I facilitated in Tbilisi, Georgia. Although the ethical issues are more widely discussed in Section 7.4, it is important to mention that all people and situations described in this book have been anonymised and consented to when possible. I trained in Georgia as a part of an international gestalt training institute that started one of the first ever training centres for gestalt therapy in the Caucasus. Gestalt therapy has been summarised as an approach that pays particular attention to five explorations: *responding to the situation, interrelating, embodying, self-recognising,* and *experimenting* (Parlett, 2015). In its essence, gestalt therapy focuses on the embodied co-creation of each situation. It starts with the here-and-now *response to the situation* that is inevitably *embodied* and *interrelated*; it invites us to *self-recognise* and to *experiment* with what is new or familiar. Although the five explorations are continuously entangled and changing, I will apply them to different aspects of this group as it was happening.

> The group I facilitated was truly international with the trainer being Polish and members coming from Armenia, Azerbaijan, and Georgia. There was an interpreter translating into Russian and even before coming there, I wondered how the group members would feel speaking in the language of a country that dominated this region for years. This was mirrored in my shame that my Russian is so limited and that I would use English, a language popularised through physical and cultural colonisation as another form of dominance.
>
> The training institute where I work offers certification from the European Association for Gestalt Therapy and so our four-year training is based on their requirements. Throughout the training, the trainee therapists are obliged to experience over 200 hours of personal development. In the United Kingdom, this means an hour of therapy per week in each year of the training, but in Georgia at that time they did not have enough gestalt therapists that could provide

this; therefore, trainees are required to have at least 50 hours of Skype therapy and three personal development groups lasting 50 hours each. I was invited to facilitate one of these groups that lasted for ten hours a day for five days. The brief I received was that although it is the third year of their training, members of this group have not started to organise personal therapy via Skype. I had some fantasies that perhaps they could not afford it or did not give themselves permission to access the support.

I decided to start the first day gently by getting to know the group and introduced exercises where they could notice what they sensed in their bodies as they reconvened as the whole group. My aim was to make visible any possible conflicts within the group and start building relationships with each of the individuals. However, after the first day, I did not have a sense that I knew anyone in this group. In the evening in my hotel room, I took a pen and paper, wrote the names and started to gather information about each of the participants. I was aware that I missed clarity about each of them and the group as a whole. I also felt some irritation that they seemed not to be forthcoming enough. What situation was I responding to?

On the second day, one of the participants added to my sense of irritation when he made several generalised statements mainly about God and life, but did not seem to want to engage on a more personal level. I suggested that he looked at all the people in the room one by one and noticed what he felt in his body (embodying and experimenting). It was a pleasant experience for him, but with one individual he noticed slight tension that we decided to focus on (interrelating). He said: "I don't think she likes me as I am Azerbaijani and she is Armenian". I noticed that the group became silent and observed them carefully. I had heard about the Nagorno-Karabakh region military conflict somewhere in the news before, but had never discussed it with people from the countries affected. I inquired how many people in the group were personally affected by this, and some group members made some bitter comments and there was a palpable sense of unease spreading within the group. Usually, I would suggest that at this stage we build more support in recognising the challenging feelings this topic brings, but at that time, I decided to follow the momentum and what I perceived to be a lack of personal sharing (self-recognising) so far in the group and suggested that people who were affected by this conflict sit in the middle of the group together and share personal stories. At this time, the whole group started to speak in five different languages, my interpreter looked confused and stressed, and a Georgian member of the group left the room shouting in English: "If someone tortured your father, then you would not like to look them in the face". I requested loudly and clearly that they return to their seats and speak slowly so that we can listen and understand each other. I assured them that it was a difficult topic and that is why it required special consideration and time. I requested that they do not engage in dialogue at this stage or a discussion about who is right or wrong, but for the next 30 minutes to talk only about how the war has affected them. I suggested this restriction to enhance the safety as I could see how upset they were and remembered my sense of irritation that I imagined was related to their sense of irritation with each other (responding to the situation).

The Armenian and Azerbaijani trainees sat in the centre and one by one shared their stories. Each of the stories was moving and deeply personal. Men went to the battlefield and never returned; their bodies were never found. Women were struggling to raise the children in post-communist blocks without fireplaces or any fuel to warm them in snowy winters. Threat, terrorism, rapes. Their universal meaning brought a sense of unity to the group that reached far beyond the cultural and political divisions. The person who left the room upset returned to notice these changes and the deep sense of unity and empathy in the group, and soon he and other Georgian group members noticed their own trauma (self-recognising). At that time, he was living in Ossetia and along with his family, experienced extreme cruelty when, in 2008, Russian soldiers took over that part of Georgia. We spent the whole remaining time processing the effects of trauma and its embodiment, noticing how many of the group's behaviours – for example, a sense of detachment from the group – are linked with their war and post-communist history.

Although gestalt therapy cannot be explained in written form as it is a therapy of experience, the above section shows what the work may look like. Gestalt therapists focus on here-and-now contact that is already structured by past experiences and current political dynamics. By careful observation and felt sense of the intricacies of contact, therapists and clients are able to become aware of the way they structure that contact and increase the freedom with which they relate.

Working with this group, I was often reminded of my father, his German upbringing in wartime and post-war Poland, in the ability I saw in myself to stay in the middle of the conflict and get two sides to recognise each other and discuss their differences. The internal Polish-German dialogue that I often have in my head (see Section 2.2.1), the war trauma my parents experienced, as well as my upbringing in communist Poland helped me to be closer to this group and to the problems they presented. Before I move on to introduce my family and the research methodology that was a basis for this book, I will discuss the need for this book in gestalt literature and research.

1.2 Who is this book for?

It is easier to describe what this book is *not* rather than who is it for. This book is not an introduction to gestalt therapy or a comprehensive guide on how to work with the themes of sexuality, masculinity, and culture. It is, however, an invitation to dialogue, discussion, and disagreement, not for the purpose of finding truth, but of exploring the perspectives that underpin the way we think, embody, and subsequently work with therapy clients. Although some learning is necessary to build dialogue with diverse groups of people, the hardest lesson in diversity is to be able to step out of our privileged self into seeing our worldview as just another perspective. This is what this book offers: just another perspective that may challenge or confirm some readers' beliefs, but most of all will show how theories, diagnosis, and engagement with therapy clients are a result of a perspective that is moderated by cultural and individual dynamics. Every relationship is different, every therapist has a different history, but we all have embodied social and cultural processes described in this book. Xenophobia, homophobia, sexism affect all of us; however, we will have different responses to them and different ways of embodying them. Various situations will call us out to explore these processes, and this book shows how dismantling a prejudice is an intimate, embodied, phenomenological process.

While this book does not aim to fill a specific gap in gestalt research, there are areas in which my thesis could potentially impact gestalt therapists' practices, their trainers, and their clients. In my career as a gestalt therapist, I have found only one article that studies the connection between culture and embodiment in gestalt therapy (Clemmens and Bursztyn, 2005). With limited literature on masculinity (Novack, Park and Friedman, 2013), sexuality (see literature reviews in Chapter 3), and social responsibility (see literature review in Chapter 2), this book ventures into areas that have not received a lot of attention in gestalt literature.

Furthermore, this book is a detailed case study of becoming a gestalt therapist. Most of the case studies presented in the gestalt literature cited in this book are abbreviated and so do not allow a full study of the therapeutic process. My work will therefore not only provide a more detailed case study of a therapy, but also of the life of a gestaltist, starting from childhood and then analysing the impact of adult experiences and training. The research will inform trainers and students of gestalt therapy how I have experienced and how I have interpreted parts of culture, which includes the culture of the training. Furthermore, using an autoethnographic methodology will enable me to critically analyse gestalt therapy as a culture, thus gaining insight and offering criticisms which may allow gestalt therapy to incorporate new knowledge or perhaps even to change.

This book is a tribute to my heritage that integrates my embodied experiences with my professional practice. Both are examined critically through cultural and political lenses but, before doing that, I introduce my family. One of the reasons why I show my personal perspective is to allow the reader to become aware of my bias and of how I construct the theories in this book through the lenses of my own journey – that of the personal and political hurts that created "me", the author of this book.

1.3 Introducing my family

My family is relatively small, a nuclear family with two parents and two children: a cis boy and a girl (see Figure 1.1). In further chapters, I refer in more detail to

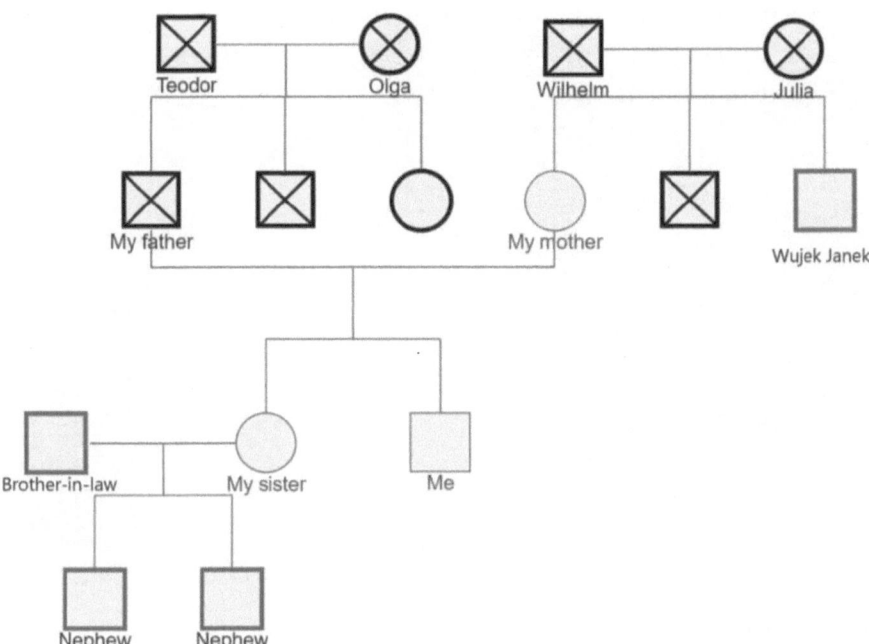

Figure 1.1 Family diagram

my father, my mother, my sister, and *wujek* (uncle) Janek. Although some of them will be separately introduced within the text, here I will present a general overview of the whole family, each of them individually as well as the interviews that I had with my mother and sister.

My mother was born during the Second World War in the territory that was incorporated into the Third Reich, Germany; thus, officially this territory was not under occupation. Coming from a working-class family, she was the only one to graduate from university, in law, in the 1960s. She met my father ten years later when she was visiting a friend working in a court in Kłodzko, where my father managed a historic archive. My father was born in 1933 as a German in Eastern Prussia. He learned Polish when the border changed and later graduated in history with many political difficulties: imprisonment and a subsequent long-lasting illness.

The quote that follows is from the interview with my mother and further introduces my family dynamics, providing an outline of the issues discussed in the interview:

> [My mother] When you were a teenager you said to me that I did not love you. I took you on my knees and said that you can blame me for everything,

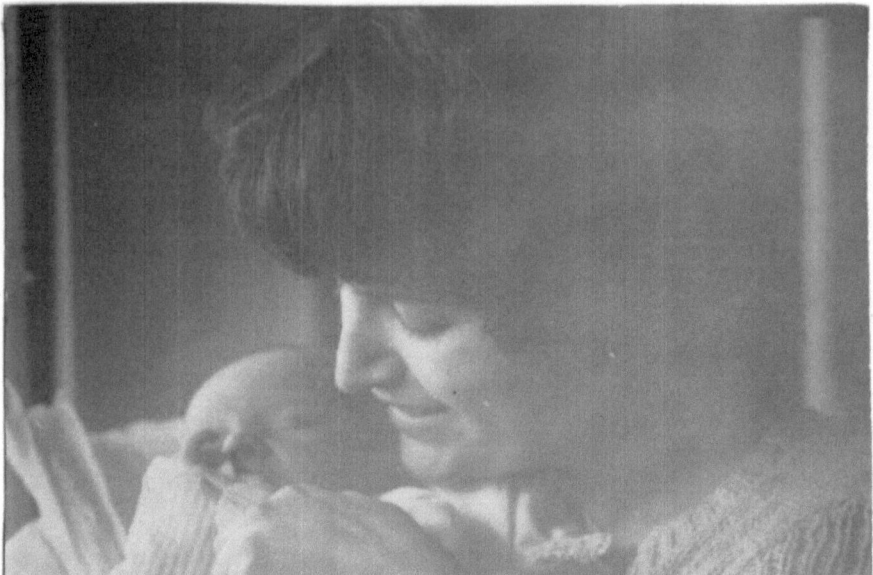

Figure 1.2 My first ever photo – mother holding me
Source: Personal photograph.

that I can admit to everything, but not that I have not loved you; this is simply impossible. I say only that I did not know how to deal with you. There are no books that say how to deal with kids at this age. You see, you wanted to go to see this therapist and your father was absolutely against it. He thought she was a witch and you should not. I did not know. I knew you were suffering, so maybe this could help or maybe not, but I gave you money and allowed to you to go since you wanted it so much. I don't know if I did the right thing, but I wanted [what was] good for you. I always had this feeling to compensate you in money or clothes, to reward you for the childhood that you didn't have. I always thought that a childhood should not look like this. I always had a poor home, but my father and mother were normal. I have only seen my father drunk twice, and this was on the 1 May.

This is how the interview started. My mother seemed defensive and scared of being judged in the process of this research. She initially blamed my father, who overused alcohol, rather than inquiring in a non-blaming way into her own circumstances. She still remembered when I blamed her as a teenager, and this interview was an opportunity to reconcile and discuss issues that we both hid for a long time (see Section 7.4.2). Her reference to Labour Day shows the cultural interconnection between communism and alcohol consumption.

My father died in 2004. I will not put words into his mouth, but I wonder what his version would be of their marriage and our family. In the interview with my sister, we reaffirmed my sense that when our father was at home sober, it was safer than when we were alone with our mother. He brought calmness and respect to our home. He also taught me how to pay attention to prejudice and to value diversity, which then shaped how I think and structured this text (see Section 2.2.1). For me, he was absent (see Section 3.2.3), as for various reasons he withdrew from the family during my early years, and I used to hold a lot of anger and upset for this abandonment. Figure 1.3 shows my father as a slightly extravagant person for the 1980s situation in a communist country. One of the very few hot countries we could go to after a lot of bribing was Bulgaria, and so we took a long train journey and spent holidays there on a couple of occasions.

My sister is almost four years older than myself. After completing a degree in anthropology, she carried on to study gestalt therapy. We argued a lot when living together in our childhood, but then found a unique connection that sometimes causes sibling envy in our friends. The interview with her turns on occasion into an interview with me (see Section 3.2.3). In the interview, she disclosed both love and struggle in relationships with our parents and agrees with my mother on how sad and difficult our childhood was (see Section 7.4.2)

Psychotherapy clients sometimes ask if there is a point in talking about the difficulties of the past, and similar questions can be asked around this research.

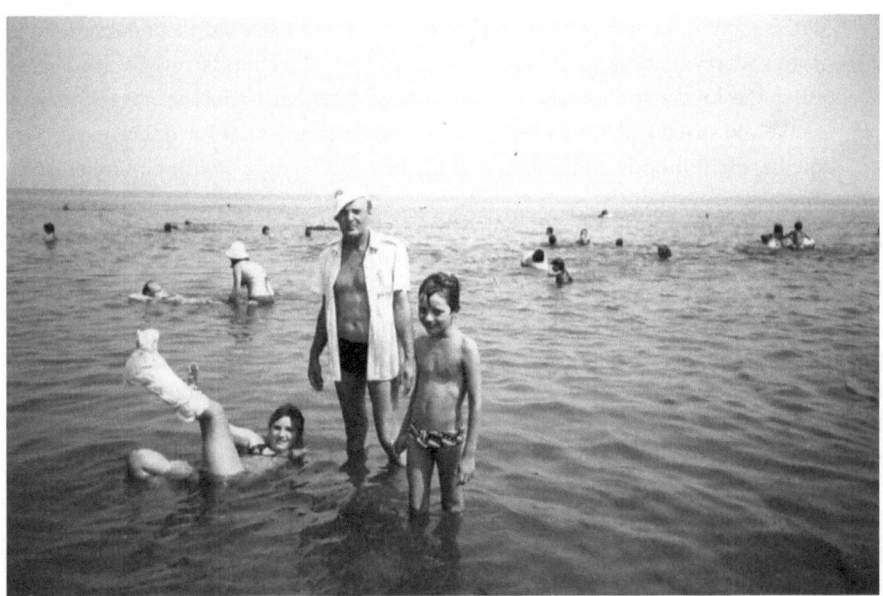

Figure 1.3 My father, my sister with a broken leg, and myself during holidays in Bulgaria, 1987

Source: Personal photograph.

I think I would not have had the courage to become so visible if I had not been introduced to and supported by autoethnographical methodology.

1.4 Research methodology

The phenomenological method in gestalt therapy focuses on embodied experiences that inform us about the co-emergent situation (Yontef, 2009), ie we feel or in other ways experience what is emergent in a situation, as happened with the Georgian training group described earlier. It is through our bodies that we notice subtle changes that happen between us. Some gestalt trainers believe that our feelings are abstractions of embodied processes (Clemmens, 2010), meaning, for example, that our sense of feeling sad could be a result of sensing some movement within our body.

> In my personal therapy, I noticed that I breathed in a way that did not support my loud speech (a condition that still occurs in moments of stress); my voice was quiet, unconfident. It reminded me of my father, who did not want me to be loud as he found me too provocative, saying things that should not be said. He himself was arrested for organising a students' protest at his university in communist Poland in 1957 and imprisoned for a year. My grandfather was arrested for collaborating with Germans, the other grandfather for being a member of the anti-Russian national liberation army, my uncles for trading in communist Poland. All the men in my family have been imprisoned and I started to understand my father's worry that my voice was too loud and clear. In contrast, my British therapist spoke loudly and clearly and she noticed how her imperialistic tendency is to take the space and not to feel guilty for doing that. We sat for hours, exploring how her British body and breath met my post-communist Polish embodied self.

The situation presented in this example took place early in my training and sharpened my interest in studying the connection between the body and culture. Looking for a methodology that would embrace the inseparable connection of *soma, psyche,* and *ethno,* I decided to use autoethnography as it is a highly personal, phenomenological study of culture. Autoethnography encourages the researcher to attend to embodied personal data that are embedded in the cultural and relational matrix (Allen-Collinson, 2013). It is a method that starts with embodiment or, more precisely, self-narration of an embodiment, that produces unique insights into relationships, cultures, and politics. By attending to the individual and insider, it provides an in-depth analysis of the cultures that produce certain embodiments; but what particular methods would best illuminate this process?

Each research methodology favours different tools that are practical ways of collecting data. While some research methodologies focus on surveys or randomised control trials, autoethnographic research studies are frequently based on three types of data: field notes, personal documents, and interviews (Anderson and Glass-Coffin, 2013, p. 65). A mixture of these data types is presented next together with justifications for why I chose each of them.

- An autobiography of embodiment and culture – I wrote a detailed autobiography that included a history of my family before I was born. It created a framework for the remembered moments from my childhood and adult life and it includes:
  - a family diagram – this enabled me to have an overview of the main relationships within my family and will provide a guide for the reader;
  - family photographs – to illustrate memories, create openings for interviews (see section on interviews that follows), and improve the intimate, evocative character of the project.

- A research journal – I kept a journal where I documented the research journey and experimented with writing about my current and past embodiment. It includes:
  - reflections on informal meetings with psychotherapists, clinical supervisors, mentors, and with other people who have had an impact on my journey. This helps to broaden my understanding of the possible ideological influences on my development as a body practitioner;
  - commissioned figure drawings by Anna Taterka depicting the embodiment of situations and states, as described in my autoethnography; these assist in illustrating my autobiography, research journal, and possibly the interview transcripts and help to bridge the gap between verbal and non-verbal communication.

- Individual unstructured interviews with my mother and sister – by coming back to my closest family, I created intimate accounts of our relationships, but also changed the relationships in the process. This gave me a greater insight into my own memories and accounts of some events.

The autoethnographic descriptions presented in this study were generated by focusing on embodied sensations and experiences. I first recorded them using the methods explained earlier, then I analysed these experiences using a particular data analysis strategy.

We all have different philosophies that we apply, and when undertaking a detailed research study, it is important to spell out what philosophies guided me through the process of writing. I applied a synthesis of Gadamer's hermeneutic phenomenology (2012) and Deleuze and Guatarri's assemblages (1987). Hermeneutic phenomenology focuses on how our embodied prejudices are uncovered through dialogue and how this very same dialogue is the best way to address them. The assemblages or *multisensory assemblages* (Renold and Mellor, 2013) encourage all voices, including the silent and, indeed, absent ones, to be heard and given space. My intention was to be able to write this book without losing the diversity of the embodied experiences, sensations, and the literature. Similarly, in the structure of this research study, as I discuss next, I paid attention to how to select the philosophies, methodology, and data that allow for the interplay between embodied sensation and collective experiences.

1.5 What is in this book?

This book is an outcome of a detailed research study that was a basis of my doctoral thesis at the University of Brighton. I have decided to present chapters on sexuality, masculinity, and culture first and leave the philosophical and methodological consideration for later chapters for readers who have an interest in philosophy and research.

The following four chapters are explorations of my recent life as an embodied gestalt psychotherapist within the social, cultural, and political field. The chapters consider the use of collective gestalts in gestalt therapy, but also enable the critical autoethnographic exploration of my own practice and gestalt therapy.

Chapter 2 contains a description of my experiences from my training and psychotherapeutic practice. It is where collective gestalts are first defined. I advocate for the efficacy of large groups as creative practices, which can lead to an increased awareness of social and cultural prejudices. I present an example of working through my own prejudices towards my own nation as an exploration of how my family situation, even well before I was born, had a direct impact on my current worldview and cultural prejudices.

In Chapter 3 I track my journey from little boy to male adulthood through a number of challenging situations and therapeutic practices that shaped my gender identity. This chapter offers insights into the negotiation of masculinities in communist and post-communist society, and explores my transition to the UK context. In it, the themes of sexual transference and hegemonic masculinity start to emerge.

Further development on the theme of the role of the erotic in psychotherapy takes place in Chapter 4, which I start from a discussion of my own heteronormativity. This creates a challenge to some current and past heteronormative practices, and points to a lack of sufficient discussion on queer theory in current gestalt therapy training and literature. The personal journey takes me to my childhood and adolescence, where I explore aspects of how my sexual orientation was formed. Reversing the old focus in psychology and psychotherapy on difference (over-researching LGBTQI communities, blackness, or disability as a way to 'other' them), I look at how heterosexual identity is formed and share my journey of deconstructing my identity through personal therapy, clinical supervision, and experiences of working with clients.

Chapter 5 refers to my initial training in gestalt therapy in Poland, followed by an exploration of my current practice as a British gestalt psychotherapist. It provides further comparison between the two cultures, Polish and British, that have been formative to my embodiment. The chapter includes a reflection on the hurt that has led to my choice in terms of my therapeutic method. That experience and my subsequent choices could be compared to the Greek myth of Chiron who, wounded by a poisoned arrow, spends his whole life researching remedies.

Although the chapters presented in this book are linked to my early life and even to the life of my family before I was born, the majority of my autoethnographic descriptions here include reflections on my current psychotherapeutic practice.

The following two chapters are theoretical. They introduce philosophies that were behind the research considerations as well as the methodology itself. Agential realism (Barad, 2007), presented in Chapter 6, is a modern post-structuralist philosophy that accentuates the unity of the physical, intellectual, and cultural. It is a useful basis for autoethnography, described in Chapter 7 as a proposed research methodology for gestalt therapists. That same chapter includes methodological and ethical considerations that could be insightful to all people considering writing autobiographically in psychotherapy.

All of the chapters in this book refer to the wider social, political, and economic environment and their relationship with and impact on gestalt therapy, heteronormativity, and cultural prejudices. They also take on an in-depth critical exploration of gestalt therapy practices and theory, which includes psychotherapeutic practices which may actually be harmful to clients. Finally, I offer an invitation to apply critical queer thinking in gestalt therapy theory and suggestions on how to include collective gestalts in current gestalt therapy theory and practice (see Chapter 8).

This book is an account of studying my own experiences, in particular my bodily sensations within a particular perspective-horizon (Gadamer, 2012). Writing each chapter began from an embodied experience and phenomenological *epoché* (attempt to suspend beliefs and assumptions) to attend to bodily sensation as felt through breath, body, and movement. An autoethnographer, Allen-Collinson, believes that *epoché* is "about approaching the phenomenon, as far as possible, with an open, enquiring, questioning attitude of mind and being reflexive and self-critical vis-à-vis my own preconceptions" (2011, p. 18). This attitude was my guide throughout my training and beyond, and opened possibilities for the experiences I had in large groups during my training. Large groups were one of the most impactful part of my training in gestalt therapy and provided the basis for collective gestalts, which I introduce in the following chapter.

Chapter 2

Defining the collective gestalt
What I have learned from large groups

In this chapter I introduce and define "collective gestalts" as having a different structure and way of embodying than "unfinished gestalts", a term usually applied to family dynamics or direct experiences from our past. Collective gestalts happen beyond the scope of our control, sometimes even before we were born, yet we actively participate in how they are collectively remembered and lived through. We embody them and, no matter how much we would like to, we are unable to be neutral towards them. The experiences within this chapter are my personal examples of attending large groups in my training.

2.1 Introduction

The "large group" component of my training was one of the most powerful modules I attended when completing my degree in psychotherapy. Through this chapter, not only do I give tribute to the learning I gained, but I also analyse the literature on large group work and social identity theory to suggest further developments in gestalt therapy. I introduce the term "collective gestalt" to describe the unfinished situations that affect whole societies and cultures and describe their nature as dialectic, meaning both dialogic and contradictory.

It is hard to imagine what a large group is without experiencing one. Usually, between 50 and 100 people sit in a circle for an agreed period of time (see Figure 2.1). Although some large group practitioners believe a large group should have at least 30 participants (see Table 2.1), smaller groups of over 18 participants are also considered as they still enable similar dynamics. There is no upper limit to large groups; however, in my experience, there is a difference when microphones have to be used or when participants can speak without them. Every large and small group brings about inherent power dynamics. Although lack of microphones democratises the process as everyone can speak when they need to, it also enables people with a louder voice and higher vocal confidence to take over the discussion.

There are various psychotherapeutic modalities that facilitate large groups. To my knowledge, there is only one large group which remains specific to gestalt therapy and meets regularly. This chapter focuses, then, on experiences from this particular group. Other gestalt large groups were used to deepen democracy

Table 2.1 Comparison of opinion on the number of people in large groups

	Large group	Median group	Small group
De Maré, 1991	30+	18–30	
Main, 1975	20+		
Schneider and Weinberg, 2003	30–35+		9–15
Turquet, 1975	40–80		
Anzieu, 1984	25–50		8–12

(Lukensmeyer, 2013) or within organisational settings (Harris, 1994). However, this chapter describes only the first day of the work; thus, it focuses solely on the formation of the group.

Large groups have also been organised and researched in: *psychoanalysis* (de Maré, Piper and Thompson, 1991; Kreeger, 1975; Schneider and Weinberg, 2003); *large-group awareness training* (Finkelstein, Wenegrat and Yalom, 1982); *process-oriented psychology* (Mindell, 1995); and *coaching* (Bunker and Alban, 1997, 2006; Emery and Trist, 1960; Katz and Kahn, 1966).

To my knowledge, current large groups include: British psychoanalytic groups (i.e. The Group Analytic Society and The Tavistock Institute), large-group awareness training that seems to have lost popularity in the 1990s (Forsyth and Corazzini, 2000), and the process-oriented psychologists' biannual "WorldWork" (Mindell, 1995). Business coaches often use large group dynamics when working with larger organisations, utilising coaching strategies such as SimuReal, Open Space Technology, Work Out, Whole-Scale Interactive Events (Bunker and Alban, 1997), The World Café, and America*Speaks* (Bunker and Alban, 2006).

In general, there are three types of large group set-ups (Foulkes, 1975, pp. 41–47):

- Problem-centred – organised to tackle a certain problem, eg to discuss and agree on a major change in the management strategy of a company
- Experience-centred – focusing on the moment-to-moment experiences of participants
- Therapy groups – almost not in existence any longer, which were offered in conjunction with small psychotherapeutic groups in therapeutic communities and mental health hospitals.

In this research, I present an experience-centred group in the context of psychotherapeutic training. During my training, once a year all students and faculty of the Gestalt Centre London attended a five-day residential away from London. When I was a member, there were, on average, 70 students and seven facilitators attending the residential group, coming from two years of counselling and five years of psychotherapy training courses. The residential was mandatory for all students.

Content-wise there were three types of activities offered during the residential: large groups, home groups, and experiments.

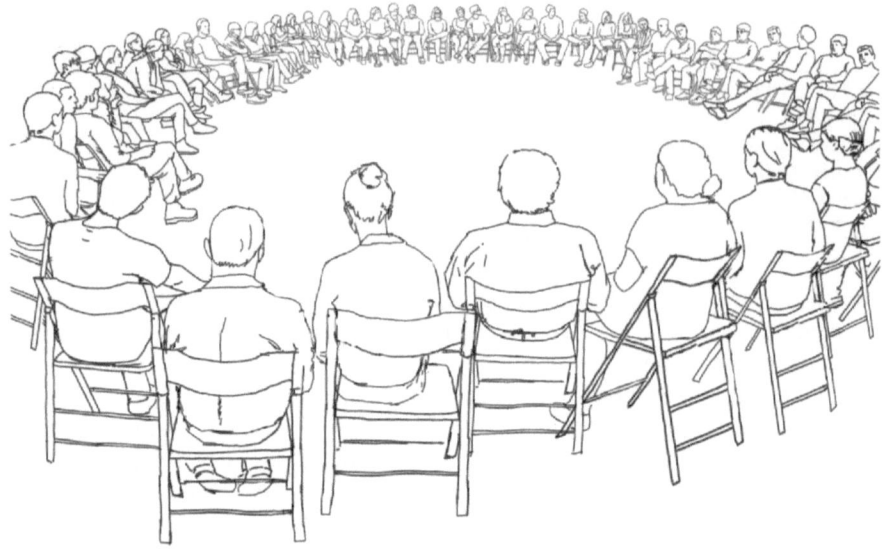

Figure 2.1 Large group session
Source: Anna Taterka (2017e).

During the large groups, all the attendees would sit, usually in a circle, with no explicit structure, except for the schedule of groups itself. When almost 80 had arrived, it was time to start. We would usually begin with a period of silence. I remember at first experiencing a profound fear during these moments, a lack of clarity as to what to say or even why I was there at all; but with time, the group was working better, and I felt more clarity and more settled. The tutors who facilitated this process made limited interventions; their main aim was to raise awareness (Yontef, 1993) of large group processes to the students.

Frequently, participants were invited to meet in subgroups, ranging from their home group (students attending the same year of training) to those based on common themes. Separate rooms were booked for these occasions.

"Experiments" at the residential were structured to include all participants who were working on a particular task together – see an example of such an experiment in my second autoethnographic example (Section 2.2.2).

2.2 Embodied dialectics

To show my personal and theoretical journey, I have included two autoethnographic experiences. Personally, the journey has been a search for cultural and political identity, which I was challenged to discover through my large group participation. Theoretically, the journey has led me to suggest that gestalt therapists consider attending to collective experiences as differentiated from individual ones, and that they hypothesise the dialectic character of these experiences.

2.2.1 Belonging in my first group – collective identity

During a large group session at the five-day residential, another student, not from my year group, says something about her struggle as a Polish woman. Three other Polish students offer support in response, and I say without much feeling that I am also Polish, and I share her struggle. What I say feels rather automatic, but I don't pay much attention to this. During the break, some of these Polish group members come over, and we exchange names. I then notice my own year group exiting through the hallway, so, I make an excuse to the Polish women and go to find my group. The following day I do not find much time to talk to the Polish people I have met. They seem to have bonded and are having a lot of fun together. One of them starts the next large group session by saying to the group how much he is enjoying this new found Polish "contingent". I then find myself wondering, would he have enjoyed it if he were gay? I notice that my imagination paints the Polish group as a rigid group of intolerant Catholics. Soon, however, this image I hold begins to fade. I realise that they seem like a genuine bunch of nice, open, future counsellors and therapists, who are of Polish origin. My ambivalence between wanting to join the group and my fear of being close to them turns into a struggle. I begin wondering why I had been so quick to judge them so harshly. The theory of internalised oppression comes to my mind, but soon I am also reminded of my father, telling me once to be wary as to whether the Catholic girl I was dating was a tolerant person, as he felt often they were not. He was from a German family who refused repatriation to Germany after the border changed in 1945. Not only was he bullied because he had come from the country which was disgraced after the Second World War, but also because he had an accent and was a Protestant. Other children called him Luther, as a taunt.

Thinking about this now, the penny drops, and I find myself flooded with tears and not able to sit in my chair.

I am surprised, on looking up, to see Polish people around me offering support. This brings a whole other wave of tears. I think, these are my people – the third wave of tears comes – this is why I emigrated.

Some of these feelings were buried deep inside me, and I certainly did not allow myself even to consider the degree of strangeness I had felt in Poland. As this experience came to me after many years of individual and group psychotherapy, I started to wonder how much the size of the group had become the *enabling solution* (Whitaker, 2001). I needed to attend to it. Some psychoanalytic writers state that large groups are qualitatively different experiences in comparison to small groups and also to individual therapy (see de Maré, Piper and Thompson, 1991).

Reflecting on how large groups affected my experience of my national identity, I have realised that belonging to a collective is an important part of a healthy functioning life and that large groups offer a unique opportunity as they bring about insights about such belonging. A short summary of the literature that bridges the sociological and psychological views of collective identities such as social identity theory, psychoanalysis, gestalt therapy, and theories on collective trauma will follow.

These processes were researched by a social identity theorist Tajfel (1981). It is not my intention to present social identity theory with all its complexity here; hence, I will not differentiate between sociological and psychological understanding of social identity theory (see Simon, 2004; Deaux and Burke, 2010).

According to Levine and Hogg (2010, p. 798), social identity theory is based on three separate theories:

- Social categorisation (Turner, 1987) – how we divide groups into categories
- Social comparison – how we associate value with each group
- Social identification – how we act in accordance to our classifications of a group.

Two analytic concepts bring similar hypotheses. First is the *"group self"*, as described by Kohut (1976, pp. 420–421). The "group self" meant the new, almost distinct quality a group-as-a-whole has or creates. Volkan developed a concept of the large group identity, defined as: "the subjective experience of thousands or millions of people who are linked by a persistent sense of sameness while also sharing numerous characteristics with others in foreign groups" (2001, p. 81).

Field theory in gestalt therapy (Parlett, 1991) states that we are all part of an interconnected environment. However, this seems rather vague compared to what I have experienced in the group described in this chapter. Although gestalt therapists would agree that distinct wholes (for example, society or culture) could be treated differently from the sum of their parts (Koffka, 1935), little attention has been given to how collective identity originates and how, practically, to work with it. While Lee (2007) argues for intersubjective ontology in gestalt therapy, Francesetti (2015) focuses on intersubjective diagnosis, but all their examples are restricted to dyads and families. Writing about small groups, several authors distinguish the environment of the small group as something unique and distinct (Hodges, 2003; Zinker, 1977). Their scope does not, however, include larger collectives. There are also examples of gestalt therapy being applied to working within communities (Nevis and Melnick, 2009), but they hardly ever refer to our own need to belong.

Attending to my embodiment after this large group example on the five-day residential, in my personal therapy and home groups, I realised a lack in the literature of gestalt therapy that would relate to my own experiences. I certainly knew that my *embodied cultural self* (Clemmens and Bursztyn, 2005) was changed and that I had felt a lot of relief afterwards. To understand it better, I decided to enlarge the gestalt concept of unfinished gestalts (unfinished business that holds our energy and prevents us from attending to here-and-now situations) to become *collective gestalts*. A collective gestalt is an embodiment of social, political and cultural circumstances through personal experiences. Defined in this way, it can also include memories passed through generations, either through epigenetics (Rodgers et al., 2015) or through early attachment with caregivers (Ruppert, 2008). So-called "repatriation" was an act of revenge in Poland towards Germans after the Second World War. An act of robbery and cruelty that thus far has never been acknowledged by any Polish government. Poles as well as those in the Red Army have often been afraid to admit their own war crimes, as well as wanting to avoid possible litigation for stolen lands and goods. With the current denial of the Polish government of crimes against Jews (BBC News, 2018), it is unlikely there will be any opportunity for reflection on the treatments of Germans after the Second World War. The sense of conflict I feel within myself has signs of cultural trauma. Alexander (2004, p. 1) states:

> [cultural trauma] occurs when members of a collective feel they have been subjected to a horrendous event that leaves indelible marks upon their group consciousness, marking their memories forever and changing their future identity in fundamental and irrevocable ways.

Attending to my *cultural trauma* was not only my individual experience but was also witnessed by other Poles and non-Poles when stating my truth. De Maré (1975) believed that it is not the individual that changes in large groups, but the whole society. My second autoethnographic example shows how this may happen in practice.

2.2.2 Political chairwork: towards the dialogic character of collective gestalts

During a large group in the final year of my training, we were invited to take part in an experiment. We were asked to work for the whole day in our year groups with an exception that we may send up to two "ambassadors" to other year groups. My small group was going through a lot of problems and we started to work eagerly on diversity and on our wide-ranging ethnicity, sexual orientation, and gender. A classmate of mine was deeply affected by a situation in the large group and, just as she started to cry, we heard a knock on the door. A first-year student appeared, an ambassador. She smiled a lot, sat in the chair and said that she had come to watch the "blood, struggle, and vulnerability of mature students". Hearing this, I started to feel sick. I wondered how I could protect her from the amount of aggression I was starting to feel. The group ignored her, but she kept interrupting. The anger

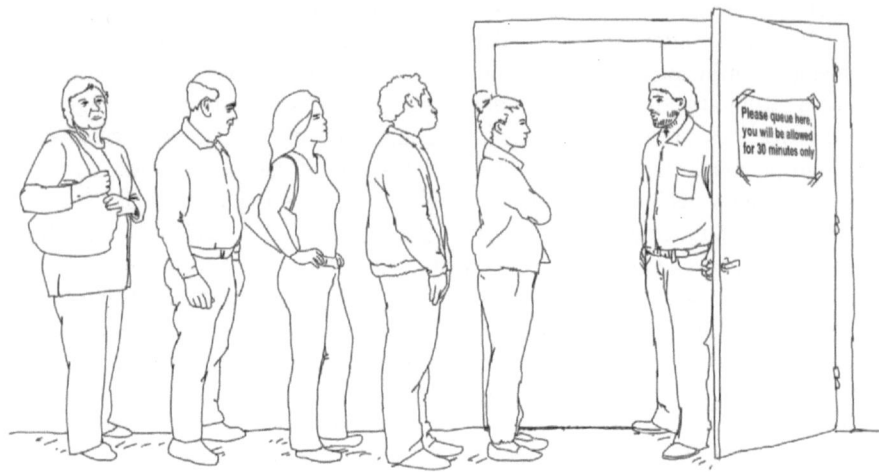

Figure 2.2 Waiting for admission to the "cool" group
Source: Anna Taterka (2017j).

the group felt towards her brought us closer, and in those moments we felt very united. Finally, she left, but was followed by another two students wanting to join. Whenever we started to open a difficult subject, sharing tears and prejudices, there was a new face, a new need, and a lot of questions. After two hours, we decided to allow only one person at a time to join us and for a maximum of 30 minutes each. When I left for lunch, I noticed a queue of people behind our door (see Figure 2.2). My narcissism kicked in; I thought to myself, they just wanted to hang out with the most mature students at the residential.

The following day, we returned to the large group and one of the newer students accused us of designing an immigration system. This was actually a very accurate description – indeed the queue we caused by our regulations looked like the "all other passports" queue at Heathrow International Airport, but . . . I like immigrants [and] I thought, I am an immigrant . . . so I was also shocked. Minute by minute this confusion led me to realise and understand what some right-wing party members feel or think, and I found a part inside me which opposes immigration. I found myself confused and enlightened through this experience as I opened a dialogue not only between the two parts of myself (pro- and anti-immigration), but also between the two parts of our society, and started building bridges rather than establishing borders.

This experience led me to realise the dialectically contradictory dynamic of how collective gestalts are embodied. Although it did not have a direct impact on my own beliefs about immigration, I became more able to relate empathically to people holding different political views. Instead of a bracing sensation within my body, I found more a softness, an ability to breathe. I have found that I am able to dialogue, not by taking a side in the polarity, but by coming to understand some of the needs of my so-called, political opponents. I came to realise that I hold inside myself a diversity of views, rather than having to act out one part of a polarity. Interestingly, it is my belief that such polarisation occurs not only within individuals, but also couples, groups, societies, and cultures. A collective gestalt becomes fixed when there is no support and opportunity for dialogue, not enough support to hold the diversity. I realised for me there had been no previous dialogue between my German and Polish parts (possibly because my father would have found it painful). Being an immigrant and a friend of many radical leftists, I was too scared to admit that there might be a part of me which is worried about immigration. I was becoming more radical and rejecting different views when I had no support for dialogue myself.

2.3 Attending to collective gestalts: support, hatred, and dialogue

I have described an example of how my own national and political identities were changed through the large groups I experienced. In the sections that follow, I will provide further theorisation about how I think this process happened.

In *social identity theory*, identity becomes changed in groups that shift in size: "identity change is a function of changing connectedness of identities within the social structure", writes Stets (2006, p. 105). This may explain why certain themes from my own life have only appeared in large group settings. Stets (2006) also links this process of opening towards others with an increasing awareness of multiple identities and ownership of each identity. This means that the more I was able to see myself in various identities, for example, German and Polish, the more I was able to be more open towards others. An increase in personal contact is also an aspect of large groups that contributes to changes in our own social identification (Dovidio, Gaertner and Kawakami, 2003, p. 13). Volkan gives another example of how awareness of multiple identities or categories as well as ownership can take place in large groups:

> I have repeatedly observed that when such representatives come together in a small group and are given the "task" (Bion, 1961) of discussing the conflictual relationship between their respective large groups, the issues pertaining to each side's ethnic, national, or religious identity assume primary importance, and their personal identity fades into the background. Each individual participant in the dialogue, regardless of his or her personality organization, professional or social standing, or political orientation, feels that his or her side is under personal attack and is compelled to defend their large group and become its spokesperson.
>
> (2001, p. 83)

In this example, large groups provide an opportunity for direct engagement through dialogue with people who do not share our beliefs. This concept is similar to Gadamer's view of the role of dialogue and prejudices. Gadamer critiqued Husserl's idea of *epoché*, suggesting that our social, historical, and political experiences and traditions have a direct and continuous impact on our epistemology:

> The great historical realities of society and state have a predeterminate influence on any "experience" [. . .] In fact history does not belong to us; we belong to it. Long before we understand ourselves through the process of self-examination, we understand ourselves in a self-evident way in the family, society, and state in which we live. The focus of subjectivity is a distorting mirror. The self-awareness of the individual is only a flickering in the closed circuits of historical life. That is why the prejudices of the individual, far more than his judgements, constitute the historical reality of his being.
>
> (2012, *p. 278*)

It is dialogue, starting with attention to our own prejudices, that can lead us to a greater awareness. As with Volkan's example (2001), Gadamer suggests an open engagement with difficulties. He states that dialogue "consists in not covering up the tension by attempting a naïve assimilation of the two but in consciously bringing it out" (2012, p. 305). When dialogue is significantly developed, it leads to the *fusion of horizons*. It is not a fusion as gestalt therapists may see it, in confluence (the merger of two parts), but more a fusion created out of exploring differences, inherently relational (Hycner and Jacobs, 1995). This is then in line with gestalt therapy's *paradoxical theory of change* (Beisser, 1970) that claims that people change when they give up on wanting to be someone else.

Therefore, collective gestalts are non-confluent and dialogic. This is what I call the dialectic nature of collective gestalts as they capture tension existing between different ideas, factions, and parts of society. The dialectics of Germans and Poles, conservatives and leftists, oppressors and the oppressed, constitute each of these collective gestalts. If the absence of dialogue creates a fixation, large groups provide conditions for dialogue often silenced by hate, politeness, and fear.

The classic book *Koinonia: From Hate, through Dialogue, to Culture in the Large Group* (de Maré, Piper and Thompson, 1991) explains how well-facilitated large groups can lead to a culture of dialogue. In line with Gadamer's idea of bringing out difficulties, they recognise the need for hatred and that with support, bringing this out can lead to a sense of fellowship, which they call *Koinonia*. The state of Koinonia is developed through dialogue that is learned in large groups. "The avowed and only purpose of the larger group is to enable people to learn how to talk to each other, to learn a dialogue" (de Maré, Piper and Thompson, 1991, p. 17).

As important as it is to attend to hatred in large groups, this also can trigger serious fear and anxiety (Skynner, 1975, p. 247). On occasions, it is not only difficult to stay vulnerable, but even to be able to think in groups which are focusing on a theme such as hatred. One may lose what Bion (1984) calls the ability to "think under fire". I believe there is no gimmick or short-term intervention that can bring people with prejudice towards each other quickly to attend to this. One thing I took for granted when studying at the Gestalt Centre was how many years of trust-building with the organisation my tutors and my fellow students had, which led to me feeling able to stay vulnerable and unpack my prejudices in the large groups. I already had close relationships with others in the group and that let me take greater risks. I had close friends looking and nodding from the other side of the room as I fought, dialogued, and cried. This is why the first step in discovering collective gestalts is to create support and relationships. To attend to how we relate to each other when we are getting in touch with our hatred or fear, those deeper relationships are necessary. Robine (2015, pp. 222–223) lists three steps in creating social change through psychotherapeutic encounter: access to the world lived by an Other; intersubjective relationship, connection, and belonging; and recognition. The last one can only appear when a great effort is put into creating the safety and belonging.

Furthermore, the psychotherapeutic theory that we use to explain large group processes needs to be treated as another prejudice, which needs to be dialogued as each of the therapeutic modalities brings a new form of prejudiced assemblage. Years of researching large groups, mainly from Freudian and Kleinian perspectives, led to a reduction of the groups to either nurturing or destructive (Volkan, 2001, p. 84). In WorldWork, facilitated by process-orientated psychologists, facilitators were actively encouraging hateful polarisations, whilst the recent analytic research promotes relational and intersubjective dialogue about vulnerabilities. They claim that confrontation creates insecurity in the group and is an obstacle, while empathy opens bridges (Island, 2003, p. 207). Any theoretical lenses should not be rigid or fixed; dialogue needs to be allowed not only between group members, but also to include facilitators.

2.4 Conclusion

Autoethnography seems to share the same task as large groups. "Within autoethnography, the selves of researcher and participant coalesce and our own experiences qua member of a social group are subject to analysis" (Allen-Collinson, 2013, p. 282). Furthermore, autoethnography presents an interesting contribution to current knowledge on large groups, as current research seems to ignore the personal experiences of group attendees. The first access to these experiences is phenomenological, and hence comes through our embodied experiences. In "new materialism" (see Chapter 6) the body is:

> a visceral protagonist within political encounters. We suggest not only that this emphasis on bodily processes and corporeal capacities is a notable element within some of the new materialisms but also that it is indispensable to any adequate appreciation of democratic processes.
>
> (Coole and Frost, 2010, p. 9)

Large group practitioners and researchers have either written about their experiences as facilitators (Island, 2003; Skaife and Jones, 2008; Skynner, 1975), or focused their attention on pre-structured questionnaires (Fisher, 1990; O'Neill, Constantino and Mogle, 2012). Considering the fact that often, due to immense fear and competition for speaking space in large groups, some group members do not speak at all, the lack of research focusing on personal stories, therefore, seems serious.

It is not enough to bring a large number of people to a large space to enable them to work through societal conflicts. Each successful large group encounter requires strong relationships between individuals and in communities to be present in the group; the experience of facilitators in managing safe expression of hateful or difficult emotions; and the opportunity to engage in dialogue, which is something that sometimes first needs to be learned.

Connecting my own experiences, then, to current theory on large groups, social identity, and social categorisation, I suggest there is a need for gestalt therapists to consider attending to collective gestalts in their work to study the impact of the political and social situation on the quality of dialogue and on the quality of contact with their clients. It is not just that collective gestalts shape therapeutic embodiments (see, for example, Section 4.1.1); current gestalt therapy theory does not offer sufficient language to theorise collective experiences, collective trauma, and our ways of working with these.

This is how the idea of collective gestalts arose from data and experiences in large groups. Examples presented here show the application of collective gestalts in the process of reconciliation and work with political differences in large groups. Large groups are not and should not be the only way to attend to collective gestalts in gestalt therapy. The work on my sexuality and masculinity required more intimate and tactile conditions to be addressed than large groups could offer. The following chapter shows how therapeutic choices are inevitably shaping gendered and sexualised bodies.

Chapter 3

Masculinity and male sexuality

How did my teenage years shape
the man that I am becoming?

This chapter explores the collective gestalt of masculinity. I begin by illustrating how early sexual uncertainties led me to start my therapy when I was 16 years old and then move on to discuss my experiences as a client and male psychotherapist. Masculinity, as with other identities that are in power (for example, whiteness), can be easily omitted and not deconstructed through research; this chapter is an attempt to contradict the invisible masculinity (Kimmel, 2012) and the fact that, in research, gender often means womanhood (Rosenfeld and Faircloth, 2006, p. 1). The limited literature on masculinity in gestalt therapy (Novack, Park and Friedman, 2013) discusses how to work with the client's masculinity without much inquiry into the gender of the therapist.

I explore masculinity and sexual intimacy in the context of family, relational, and cultural dynamics, focusing on the phenomenological analysis of the interplay between the body and the context. Men's sexual problems are presented as dependent on historical conditions reenacted in the current situation. That dependency deconstructs the masculine belief in individual potency that is further deconstructed by the disclosures of my own temporary impotencies. Among discussed conditions that shape my sexuality, I focus on the transgenerational transition of trauma, communism, differences between attitudes to sexuality between Polish and English psychotherapists, masculinities, and a relational approach as opposed to the individualistic thinking in medicine and psychology. This chapter portrays the embodiment of an intimate dialogue between myself in different stages of my life and the collective gestalt of masculinity.

In the following section, men's sexuality is presented through vulnerability and questions of what being a man is. Men's sexuality is not as independent as we would like to think, but is dependent on transgenerational trauma, class, and society and is fragile, emotion-based, and vulnerable. Medicine and psychotherapy are dominated by patriarchal structures that often analyse problems from the perspective of single dominant heterosexual masculinity (see Section 3.3.2). The journey of my manhood shows how different masculinities were born and lived throughout my life often in contradiction with one another.

3.1 Sexuality, paradoxical theory of change, and experimentation in gestalt therapy

3.1.1 Autoethnography: why I decided to start therapy

When people ask me why I started therapy when I was sixteen, I usually reply that I was a troubled teenager. Rarely do they enquire what I mean by this, but even less rarely do I offer an honest answer when asked.

I think I was eight when I got my first computer and that immediately provided respite and relief from the playground on my estate. I was bullied there and dreaded each time I had to pass through it to go to school or the shop. After the computer arrived, my childhood oscillated between programming, playing, and hiding in the staircase of my block (far right on Figure 3.1) when my parents got impatient with me for spending all my time indoors and forced me to go out. I imagine that they knew I was bullied and wanted me to get stronger and sort it out, while at the same time never discussing this topic with me nor talking to the parents of the boys who bullied me. I remember these moments when my mother rushed into my bedroom (knocking was not an option at that time in my home) and shouted:

– Why are you spending so much time on the computer?
– Turn it off now (she continued her monologue)
– Go out, play with other boys; be like a normal boy!

At that time, I had no choice but to leave and spend time either in the large and complicated staircases of my block or wandering round my estate looking for Przemek, a boy who had much respect from boys on the estate and who protected me when he was around. It was a mining estate where most of the families spoke Silesian, and we were allocated this flat because my mother worked in the administration of a mining servicing company. I was one of the few boys that spoke Polish without an accent and did not have much in common with other boys, maybe except for the fact that most of our fathers had an equal amount of alcohol consumption per day.

Most of the time I spent discovering various options of my Commodore C64 that was soon replaced by a PC. For those who also find geeky moments senti-mental, it was 486SX 25Mhz with 245Mb hard drive. Programming in a language called Basic was surprisingly entertaining considering that the outcome of a whole day of work could have been a ball flying through the screen. More exciting was the world of computer games where I usually impersonated a ruler of the world with soldiers calling me "my lord" (Warcraft), "master" (Dune II) or "commander" (UFO Enemy Unknown). That was a big change in my life after feeling humiliated by other boys each time I left my apartment or block and this reality, although virtual, provided compensation for most of the uncertainties in my real life.

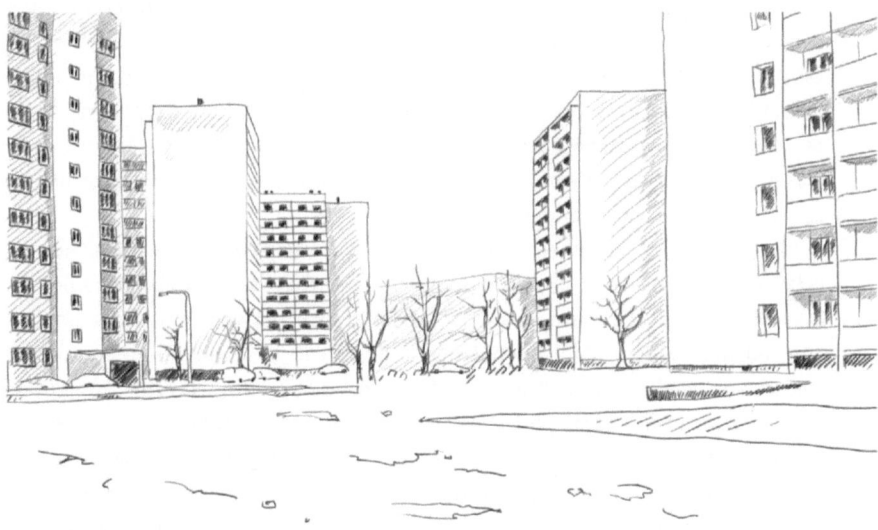

Figure 3.1 The estate where I grew up
Source: Anna Taterka (2017f).

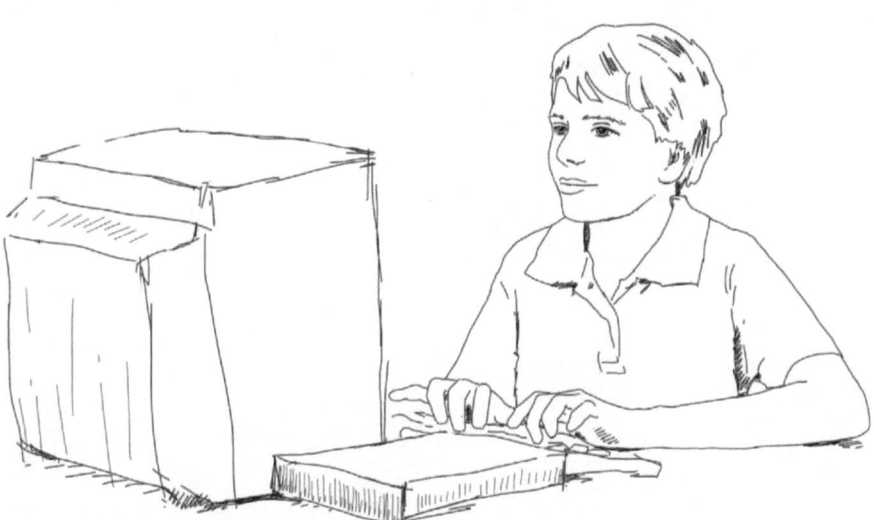

Figure 3.2 Playing and programming – 1988–1996
Source: Anna Taterka (2017h).

There is a significant difference between waiting for my father to come home drunk at night while not being able to sleep and the same experience when successfully solving a Star Trek RPG (Role Play Game) mystery, hearing my father unlocking the door at 2 a.m. and clumsily moving around the apartment. As far as I remember, my parents did not sleep in the same room and my father's room was just next to mine. I was often unable to sleep, feeling responsible for him, or at least ready to act if needed.

My only and older sister moved out when I was twelve, and since then my relationship with her has become much better. I think I felt easily overwhelmed by women who are close to me; so, the distance between my sister and me allowed me to feel that I missed her and wanted to connect. My sister (see Figure 3.3) lived in another town about two hours' drive from my hometown, and we met almost fortnightly. She brought me some books, usually American realism, John Irving, Joseph Heller, and later Henry Miller, that showed me that there was another reality that was not virtual, but also manageable. People in her books were troubled but usually found a way to enjoy their lives as well in precious moments. I was so inspired by her and the reading that against the advice of my parents, teachers, and common sense, I decided not to pursue a career in IT, but to focus on Arts, Humanities, and Languages when transferring to the high school at the age of 15.

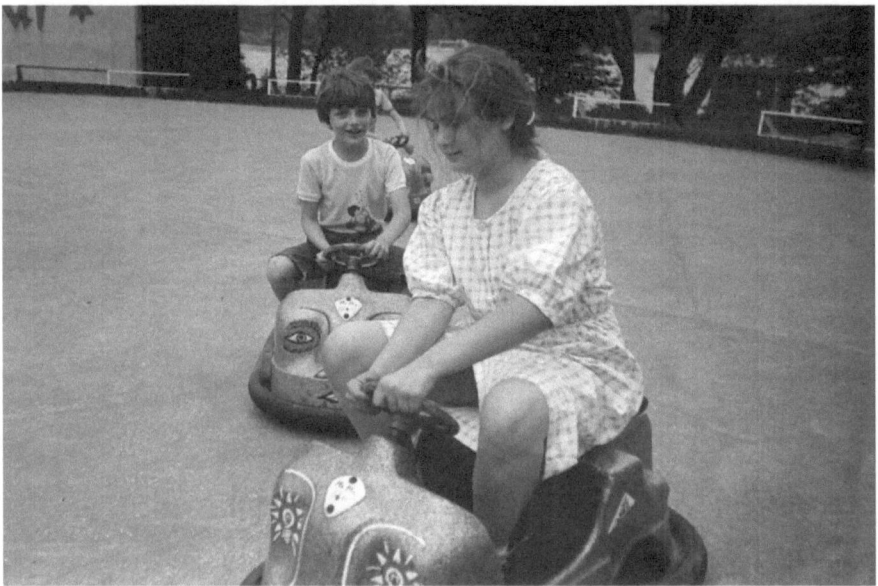

Figure 3.3 My sister and me, 1987, four years before she moved out
Source: Personal photograph.

What I also knew was that I found it very difficult to engage outside of my computer. Hearing someone speaking about computer addiction on the TV, I started to worry that I was dependent on computers in the same way my father was on alcohol. I used to go to sleep at 2 a.m. and get up at 6 a.m. to play games. When a screen turned blank before a film in a cinema, I could see an imprint of my computer screen and moving objects from a game I was playing at that time. When my mother wanted to restrict my use of the computer, I would have a tantrum until she agreed I could use it for an indefinite "a little longer". I found that the only solution was to sell it; so, I went to a local newspaper and posted an ad and sold it within the following two weeks.

It was shock therapy, but a necessary step in putting my life back on track. All of this could have led me to believe that I needed therapy, but it was not convincing enough for me to include another adult in my life. First, I did not trust them, and second, I felt I was doing fine.

In high school, I started to form some friendships and realised that most of the peers I wanted to hang out with had much more life experience than me. They had sexual experiences and romances; they also had a much more extended network of friends that knew how to give an impression of being cool. Faking or lying has never been an option for me; so instead I decided to be brave, override my anxieties and experiment with alcohol, drugs, and straight sex.

My parents felt so relieved that I had a life outside of the home that they not only completely let me do whatever I wanted, but also sponsored most of my wishes for the first two years of my high school. I attended every party and during one of the first ones we started to play a bottle game, and I ended up kissing a girl that I liked but did not adore. My first kiss was braved through alcohol, as often in my life pretending that I am more advanced than I was. A compliment from that girl that she liked the way I kissed made my heart melt, and although I fancied her best friend much more, I decided that I wanted to be in a relationship with her. It was such a beautiful experience that someone found me attractive, offering herself to me, that this feeling overrode all my preferences and fears. I also ignored the fact that she kissed me through a bottle game challenge, deliberately adjusting the bottle to kiss me and doing it in front of a group of people. She had a way of hiding her fears behind a challenge; so, a few months later instead of saying:

– Honey, I feel afraid of how it will work out between us and I feel I would like to take the next step with you ...

She said:

– Why don't you fuck me like that guy in the summer who I still remember?

My body was ready for that. I wanted to make her feel good and to prove that my first time would be as good as the first kiss, but instead I ended up with a floppy penis feeling hot and embarrassed. When viewed from a binary (yes or no) perspective, this moment of not being able to have sex is like the end of a night in a club when suddenly all the lights come up and instead of the sexy, smoky atmosphere, you realise that you are surrounded by some drugged and sweaty people and a bunch of staff and cleaners waiting to go home.

This is why I started my personal therapy.

3.1.2 Masculinity and class

The description presented earlier of my childhood isolation and anxieties will be analysed further throughout this chapter. In this section, I will focus on the class relationships within my estate that led me to question how well I fitted in the role of a man. As femininity is often felt as inscribed and almost unavoidable for women in our society, masculinity is something that needs to be earned (Seidler, 1997) or achieved (Loe, 2006, p. 27). The constant struggle of not feeling good enough to be a man and boy and having to prove it had a major impact in my childhood, and later in my adulthood. In this section, I discuss interference between the work status and schooling system.

Although critical reflections on masculinity are under-represented, there are some studies that show the relationship between masculinity and labour (Collinson and Hearn, 1996; Haywood and Mac an Ghaill, 2003; Morgan, 2004). Class creates conflictual models of masculinity (Morgan, 2004, p. 169) as the production of masculinities in capitalism locates the negotiation of manhood in the complex dynamics of society based on production and trade. The masculine polarisation into "'them' and 'us' [. . .] 'mental' and 'manual' and 'skilled' and 'unskilled'" (Ibidem, p. 170) seemed to take precedence even in a society designed on Marxist principles. My experience is that a communist system in Eastern Europe produced similar questions even though the power relationships manifested, through salaries, for example, were different. The miners on my estate earned much more than my father who, at that time, was managing libraries in my hometown, Racibórz. Miners had access to special shops where they could buy imported goods and food products that were not widely available. Furthermore, most of the national events were to celebrate their hard work and the government offered them preferential access to universities, and a vast number of holiday places and medical institutions that were not available to middle-class people, who were called, often in a sarcastic way, the intelligentsia. This shift of power was neither able to change the bitterness of workers and their children on my estate nor the middle-class attitudes towards labourers that I heard in some of the jokes made in mine and other middle-class families. The main difference between workers and management both in England and communist Poland lies in the fact that there is much higher job satisfaction amongst management, while workers treat the work as a means to an end (Collinson, 1992). This creates bitterness and a sense of being underprivileged, which led workers to form the Solidarity Union that demanded democracy and capitalism to address these difficulties. This process led to a majority of them being made redundant in the 1990s as there was less need for coal in the capitalist economy. What united workers in a communist, post-communist, and a capitalist country and differentiated them from *the* intelligentsia was the fact that they did not like their job and would not have done it if they had an alternative. The bullying I experienced on my estate was an outcome of these inequalities, with me playing into my inherited mild sense of being better and above all this. Working-class boys' aggression was an attempt to equalise this dynamic and deal with their shame dynamic (i.e. the sense that there is something wrong with them). These attitudes were reinforced through the school system.

In the 22nd minute of the interview, my mother illustrates how the class dynamic was performatively (Butler, 1993) constructed during a student camp for children of miners and other workers of the mine:

> [My mother] [The childminder] said that whenever a group wanted to do anything, you and your sister were against it. You were always insubordinate, always different and there were problems with you. You have never given up, she said, even if they hit you and you did not manage well in this children's camp; you were always insubordinate, always went against them. Maybe you were too young? The childminders said that you climbed on their knees and wanted to be cuddled. Because of your contrariness, other kids were against you and there was a show with all kids. The childminders said that you recited poetry and sang well, and Przemek mumbled something, but other kids clapped for him, not for you. You were yourself and even if they hit you, you still did what you thought was right and never subordinated.

In this example, the interplay between the privilege of my education and independence in my childhood is positioned against the aggression and need to conform with the working-class boys. Paradoxically, my lack of subordination was the only way to save my dignity and freedom even though the price was bullying, and a lack of support, evidenced by my need for closeness and support from the childminders. Similarly, at my school, boys from working-class families earned prestige by actively opposing education. Being a good student was associated with being effeminate (Mac an Ghaill and Haywood, 2011), similar to intellectual professions being named as not masculine enough (Haywood and Mac an Ghaill, 2003). Furthermore, the educational establishment sustained middle-class values, similar to Britain (Ibidem, 2003). Boys speaking with a Silesian accent were humiliated and picked on by teachers, while at the same time there was not much support for Silesians to learn Polish pronunciation. On the contrary, children from middle-class families had additional, paid private lessons with the same teachers who assessed their performance at school. There seemed to be no awareness of the growing gap between boys from working- and middle-class families except for occasional fights that led to injuries. However, at that time, teachers were quick to associate disturbances with individual children from working-class families, rather than a system unable to address the inequalities.

The earlier analysis shows the inescapable association of masculinity with class, whereas association between masculinity and sexual orientation is discussed in Chapter 4. Masculinity as a force, either social or personal, is often associated with competition for power and dominance (Bourdieu, 2001). In a communist society, these dynamics were dissociated from the relationship to wealth. It is men's sense of lack of work satisfaction (regardless of the income it offers) and boys' need to belong and be accepted for who they are that contributed to the described division earlier.

These divisions created a basis for my initial withdrawnness from social life and impacted on how anxious I felt when creating new relationships in my teen-age years. The next autoethnographic example is an account of my first therapy that started when I was 16 years old and shows how inexperienced psychothera-pists may feed into clients' early life sexual anxieties.

3.1.3 Autoethnography: first therapy

My first therapist was 32 years old and, at the time, this felt like a large age gap. During the first session, I told her what I wanted to work on, and she had a skilful way of showing me that therapy would include much more than just my sexual concerns, but it would be a review of how I was behaving in relationships with others. We started focusing on how desensitised I was, but at that time I could not comprehend why I needed feelings. I thought that people divided into two categories: those who feel are weak and there are people who can be above feelings. I was obviously striving for the latter; so, when she asked me what I felt the first time, I thought that she wanted to test if I was weak, and so I said "noth-ing". For quite a while we had a silent war as she wanted to get into my feelings without exploring my mind and I found my mind to be the safe place and wanted to cognitively understand where she wanted to take me. After some time, she gave up and eventually explained to me why I need emotions. I was more able to agree on this starting point and had many examples from the novels I read to trust these experiences.

When finally I developed enough trust to acknowledge and name some of my feelings, I realised that I had almost no vocabulary for subtleties of feelings and body sensations. Furthermore, my awareness of my body was limited, and my breath very shallow.

My therapist called herself a gestalt therapist, but now I know that she was mostly bioenergetically orientated. Although some guidance and psychoeduca-tion may have been appropriate for my age, she approached my body with the determination of a personal trainer who would guide me to grow bigger, stronger, taking much more air and space, being more in tune with my body and bolder in social interactions. The first task was to deepen my breath and to get in touch with the totality of my body; so, for the next many sessions, I was lying on a mattress, practising how to breathe and attending to feelings that emerged in this process. When a feeling emerged, she usually gave me some time to attend to it and often a cuddle if I cried.

Some practical exercises were proposed to help me to deal with my "sexual incapacity", and although I did not believe the problem to be physical as I could sustain an erection when masturbating, I thought that physical support could help me in a moment of emotional crisis.

At that time, being 17 years old (see Figure 3.4), I was not necessarily aware of how seductive I was in all relationships with women and men, and how I wanted to be both seduced and to seduce my therapist. I think I went on a mission to impress her and become a very good client. I heard from my friends that knew her personally that she was writing her final case study based on my case. Being a subject of her case study flattered me, but also indirectly linked her professional achievements with my erection, which already had a lot of other emotional pressures.

When I lost my virginity, I was a year into a relationship with Inga, who was more experienced than me, but also much more patient and open for exploration of a sexuality that we enjoyed rather than a sexuality that we had to perform. At that time, I started to be more and more rebellious about my mother's expectations

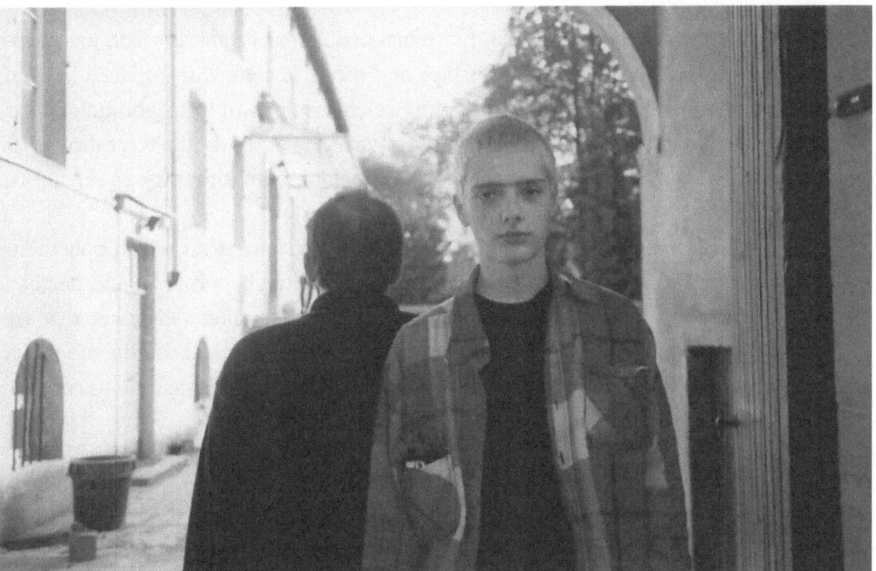

Figure 3.4 1997 – a photo from a theatre workshop, while I was wearing the 1970s jacket from my father with a Walkman with headphones in the right pocket

Source: Personal photograph.

to be a polite and beautiful boy, and so I dyed my hair (see Figure 3.4), then shaved my head, and wore the same jeans and long jumper each day. Being torn between different labels that teenagers identified themselves with at my high school, I chose Buddhism, which I understood in my teenage mind as a practice of meditation, modesty, and marijuana. I deliberately did not take care of my appearance or how well I performed at school as I did not want to please my mother or in fact any-body else. The rebellion against pleasing other people moved to my therapy where I started to be angry with my therapist for taking pride in my work. The fact that she wrote the case study based on me without taking into consideration how it may affect me led to more and more distance between us. Not wanting to please her, I did not tell her that I lost my virginity for the first few months. Only when discussing some other problems in my relationship with Inga did I mention the fact that we had sex (at that time I associated penetration with sex).

A month later I quit my therapy due to several boundary breaches. My thera-pist at that time knew my sister and my other friends. It is common practice to decline clients who are even vaguely associated with us in our private life, but my therapist had not secured my therapy in that way. It is hard to judge the first gen-eration of therapists in Poland after the collapse of communism and the quality of support and education they received. Nevertheless, this situation left me quite wounded, disappointed, and more careful in relationships with other therapists and, later, my clients.

Did this therapy help me with my sexual problems? I think it made me more confident in interpersonal relationships and more in tune with my feelings, and both facts contributed to establishing the relationship with Inga, who helped me more than any therapy. My therapy in these years helped me also to realise what I wanted to do and was a major factor in choosing psychotherapy as my future profession.

My relationship with Inga ended due to one of those reasons which only teen-agers can invent. There was a problem that I multiplied by a million and decided that in the long run it would never work. I cried for days after telling her that we would not be going out together any more. It was one of those beautiful moments I remember with my mother, who delayed our holidays to give me time to recover.

3.1.4 Sexuality, body, and change

Before I analyse further what happened in my therapy, I would like to introduce an important component of gestalt therapy that is the paradoxical theory of change. It states that clients change when they become more who they are rather than whom they think they should be (Beisser, 1970). Although my first therapist was occasionally able to adhere to this value, I was more than aware that in her eyes I needed to change, that my breathing, body posture, the amount of physical space I was taking through my body and movement, and anxiety about erections were the things that needed to change. That attitude enhanced my already felt sense that I was deficient and had to earn my masculinity. For me at that time, similar to men in Loe's study (2006, p. 36) who use Viagra: "A limp penis or absence of virility appears to symbolize death of the body as well as of manhood". In fact, the bullying, general sadness in my childhood, and even occasional suicidal thoughts at that time would not bring me to therapy, but my sense of endangered manhood would. I felt I needed to act; hence, I started my gestalt/bioenergetically orientated psychotherapy.

There is something about bioenergetically trained therapists (see Chapter 5), but also therapists coming from cultures that favour "the expansion" (the belief that taking more space is a sign of good mental wellbeing), that they want clients to grow in a certain way. In gestalt therapy, this is usually done through shaming and imposing concealed behind a phenomenological exploration of the body. For example, a therapist may say: "I am noticing how little air you take and wonder if you would like to experiment with taking a deep breath to see how you may feel". There are two innocent phrases here that under careful examination are not so innocent. Although *noticing* may be considered as a spontaneous observation of what is, it is in fact judgement, prejudice (Gadamer, 2012), an act of *Gestaltung* (Perls, Hefferline and Goodman, 2003): seeing reality through the lens of our needs and concerns. The second phrase, "wonder if you would like to experiment", is an imposition, considering the power dynamic in the therapy room. There is an implied judgement on the clients if they decline. Furthermore, there is an implied expectation in the therapy room that the therapist will be someone to give instructions, and there is an unaware pressure on the therapist to find ways to look as if they are doing something. Engaging in teaching phenomenology of the body to our clients seems to be an exercise that I find myself guilty of when I succumb to this pressure. That pressure is deeply embedded in the socially constructed hegemonic masculinity that preaches expansion and activity (rather than passivity and acceptance).

An alternative approach that follows the paradoxical theory of change would be to meet the client where that person *is*, in a relationship with us, and to explore how they embody the world from their perspective. To use the example from earlier, the therapist could have had at least two options:

Example 1

I am noticing how much I want to make suggestions to you, how I want to tell you how to breathe and how I would like you to stand . . .

a.   This reminds me of how you were bullied and of my wish to protect you
b.   I am aware that I would feel pleased if you were the way I want you to be and this surprises me
c.   I feel like I would like to take care of you as if you were very young

Example 2

I am noticing how little air you seem to take . . .

d. I have a sense that part of you wants to hide and not be seen and wonder if this is because of what I said a moment ago
e. I am aware that if I try to take that little air myself, I feel numb and somehow safe. I could imagine that you may feel unsafe with me now

These examples are not exhaustive. We can only reply to clients from the current situation we share with them; however, these are the replies that to me would feel more accepting and curious about our processes. Each of them invites us not only to explore the "enduring relational themes" (Jacobs, 2011), but also the current relational dynamics between the client and the therapist, which would have led in my first therapy to a different outcome.

In Example 1, the therapist focuses on her embodied resonance and the need to take care of the client. In my case: a. would lead to an exploration of my relationship with my sister; b. to uncover dynamics with my mother and how we recreated them in the therapy room; and c. to how I behave to make women feel concerned about me. Example 2 addressed the bullying as well as general lack of safety in a communist society that my family went through.

Although in critiquing this relational approach one may say that I am "a meaning-making therapist" who does not give enough space to what is emerging from the body, I argue that there is a considerable amount of implied judgement in the way Husserlian phenomenology is applied in gestalt therapy, and body sensations do not exist outside of the context (a further discussion of this phenomenon is presented in Section 5.2.3). All body sensations are a mixture of current and historical dynamics (Merleau-Ponty, 2005) that are being recreated within here-and-now dynamics. An example comes out in a gestalt experiment that was offered by my second therapist.

3.1.5 Autoethnography: university days – second therapy

When I started my next therapy in my early 20s, I did not complain about my lack of erection or the uncertainty. Partly in reaction to my previous therapist, my work now with an experienced female gestalt psychotherapist included looking at my sexuality and boundaries. On the boundary of my skin, I felt the enormous tension that I associated with being close to my mother and other women. A kind of burning sensation that made me feel hot and wanting to shake that imaginary something off my skin. The first thought that came to my mind was that when my mother was getting closer to me, she was usually not noticing how I might react to her. I used to call it a "kiss attack" when she just kissed and kissed my face, ignoring the fact that I did not like it. Exploring my sense of being physically overwhelmed by my mother (see interview quoted in Section 3.3.4) brought some memories from the time when I was about six and my mother used to check out my pockets. Sometimes to find a tissue or anything else, she used to feel entitled to search through the content of my pockets and often in that process I could feel her touching my genitals and feeling too embarrassed to voice my protest. Although I remember a sense of liking it, I also remember being totally frozen, unable to say anything and very embarrassed both during this situation and afterwards. If it is true that "freezing" is a component of trauma (Levine, 1997), that indicates that my sexual trauma took place much earlier. However, in my therapy during my early 20s, we focused more on how I could protect my boundaries.

The therapist suggested an experiment (Figure 3.5) in which she was reaching out with a long foam cushion to my genitals and was supporting me to voice my protest, to find clarity and push in saying no and to unfreeze at the moment when I felt embarrassed and violated. Although looking at this therapeutic work from the perspective of a psychotherapist trained in England I feel horrified at the possibility of an action in which a therapist indirectly touches the genitals of a patient, as a client I welcomed this intervention and found it very useful. The

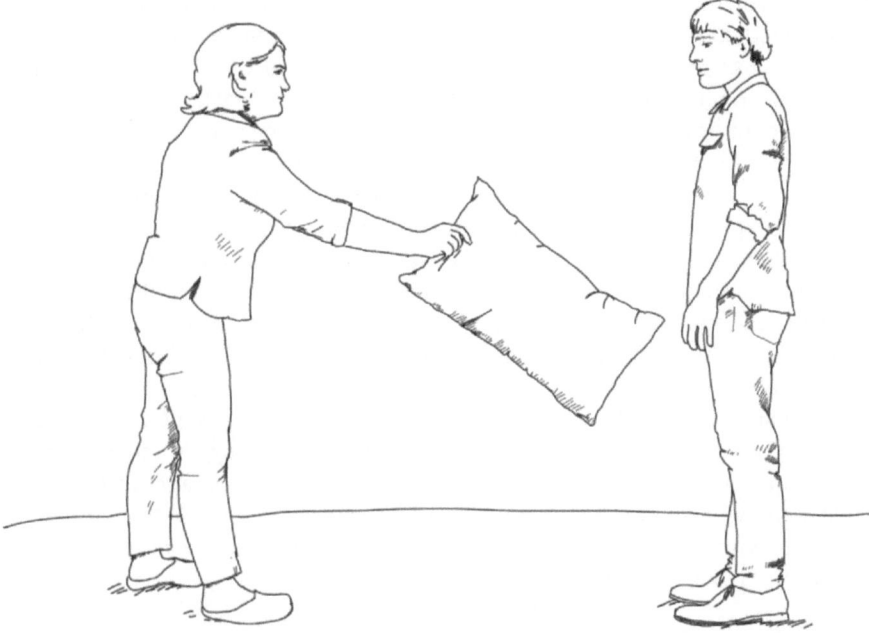

Figure 3.5 Experimenting with sexuality and violation
Source: Anna Taterka (2017b).

care the therapist took in doing it and her ability to listen made me hopeful that my boundaries would be respected and that my voice could be taken into consideration.

3.1.6 (Sexual) experimenting in gestalt therapy

Free and spontaneous experimentation has always been at the core of gestalt therapy. An experiment in gestalt therapy is a structure for exploration. It is a structure that does not reduce but enhances the dialogical nature of an encounter between the client and the therapist (Yontef and Schulz, 2013). Experiments are not planned or aimed at changing clients' behaviour, but always emergent from the context and co-designed by all parties involved. In line with the paradoxical theory of change, there are no outcomes or expectations of the experiments and whatever emerges is an acceptable outcome. Each experiment is thus an experiment into awareness, to notice what one may feel or sense, without aiming at a particular change or outcome. It is important both to remember that each experiment is always part of the therapeutic relationship, and that by not experimenting with the erotic and sexual we confirm that it is a topic not to be touched.

Earlier I described two types of experiments in my first and second therapies. While bioenergetically orientated experiments were aimed at changing the way I was embodied (both to make me bigger as well as to connect energetically with the felt sense of my genitals), the experiments offered by my second therapist explored the relational dynamic of what I felt and how I reacted to her. I imagine that I would have benefited more from the experiments suggested by my first therapist if she had included relational dynamics, for example: when do I shrink my body and when do I take more space with her? It is the interplay between personal experience and relational dynamic that experiments should seek to illustrate; hence, it is important that we take into consideration what clients communicate to us throughout experiments; how the struggle presented in the experiment is recreated in the dynamics between the therapist and the client; and what is the result of us being an observer invited into this experimentation. It is also common for therapists to struggle with relational exploration of sexuality (Renn, 2013). The therapeutic assemblage (Deleuze and Guattari, 1987) cannot and should not reduce the situation to a single individual, thereby leaving the client exposed while protecting the therapist. In fact, therapists need to be able to be vulnerable, and "vulnerability is a kind of relationship that belongs to that ambiguous region in which receptivity and responsiveness are not clearly separable from one another" (Butler, 2016, p. 25).

The erotic is inherently contagious. It creates the confusions of desire: "Whose feelings are these? Who started it? Who are you to me? Who am I to you? Where are the boundaries between desire and action?" The erotic moves not only the client but also the therapist into realms of ambiguity, ambivalence, excitement, anxiety and disgust. How can this be good for anyone? How do I contain and use my erotic countertransference as a source of information rather than a means of contagion?

(Cornell, 2003, p. 101)

The attention to the embodied resonances (countertransference) is difficult when we are affected by the societal repression of sexuality through shame and litigation. For that reason, experimentation with sexuality in therapy is an area that many therapists feel averse to. Although fear of litigation and societal prejudices towards sexuality affect the therapeutic space, it is important that sexuality and sexual experimentation are not ignored. It is important that we create the safe emergency (Perls, Hefferline and Goodman, 2003, pp. 277–289; Swanson, 1982), a state where clients and therapists are provided with enough safety to experiment with difficult emotions. Experimentation in gestalt therapy often aims to recreate here-and-now conditions that can deepen our awareness of our situation. The experiments will lose their energy if therapists are risk-averse on one hand, and may retraumatise the client if the level of risk is too high on the other hand. The mastery of a gestalt therapist lies in the way they design the experimenting on the edge of safety in line with Laura Perls' motto: "to give as much support as necessary and as little as possible" (Amendt-Lyon, 2016, p. XV).

What is allowed then, when it comes to sexuality and intimate areas? A complex range of factors that are connected to clients' attitudes towards sexuality, sexual experience, family, gender, society, and culture. When I suggest an experiment around allowing sexual feelings during my workshops for psychotherapists, I use a disclaimer that receiving an instruction from a man to explore sexuality may be difficult in itself for some of the participants due to fear of abuse beyond therapeutic boundaries.

Writing about sexual resonance in psychotherapy, Hyde gives an example of a teenage client who requests a change of therapist through an administrator before gaining enough strength to discuss her sexual dreams with the first therapist (2006). As therapists in private practice, we do not have this additional administrative support as we are the only point of contact with our clients. Most of the ethical guidance for psychotherapists promotes relational ethics, but do we, as male therapists, feel we have enough support behind our back to address sexuality with our clients as an embodied and relational phenomenon? Of course, when clients take complaints outside of the room, that usually exposes a lack of safety and relational rupture. Our fear of being unsupported within psychotherapeutic establishments and ostracised by our colleagues and friends for dealing with sexuality in therapy must have an impact on how we do or do not discuss challenging topics. The work with sexuality should not, therefore, be restricted to consulting rooms, but also psychotherapeutic supervision, peer-reviewed publications, or even political meetings where we can find support and raise awareness of this complex and necessary issue.

In the 1970s and 1980s, therapists were handing over pornographic magazines so that their clients could explore new sexual options (Maltz, 2010). However, since pornography is now easily accessible online and frequently consumed out of compulsive needs, with the internet as a medium creating long-lasting relational detachment, we need to find ways to bring our sexual dialogue forward without objectifying and removing sex from its relational context.

On the other hand, we also need to take into consideration that experiments we commonly use in gestalt therapy are already experienced as erotic, if not sexual. The use of touch which some of us offer in groups or individual work, and improvisation with space and movement, is, by definition, erotic. Otherwise, they are no longer free and spontaneous. How prepared are we to bring in sexuality as part of the discussion in the work we do?

3.2 Embodied field: the politics of the erotic

3.2.1 Autoethnography: therapy in England

About three years later, I was already based in London and getting on with my psychotherapy qualification. I then started one of the most influential psychotherapies in my life. Staying in therapy for over four years with Lesley (pseudonym) was a process where I gained the emotional stability that I so desperately needed. I found this therapist from a recommendation by a Polish institute, so I felt intrigued to work with someone who was British but also interested in exploring my culture. Although I deliberately wanted to work with someone more senior to avoid feeling attracted to that person, in the moment of fear or anxiety I still brought a lot of seduction and eroticism to the room.

Around the same time in my psychotherapy training, I was practising psychotherapy in triads (therapist, client, and the observer) almost every week with Clara (pseudonym), a foreign fellow student who was gorgeous, both physically and mentally. She taught me a lot about how to work with sexuality in the room through being very accepting of my attraction to her, open to exploring her attraction to me, clearly boundaried, and so I knew we would never take it outside of the therapy room. My longing for her was a reaching out for help, friendship, love, self-acceptance, and control. I thought that only if she found me attractive, her heart would open to me; furthermore, that only through seducing her would we be close and intimate. My self-worth and self-acceptance were also at stake as I had learnt to believe that I earn these through other people, mostly attractive women and, of course, to seduce her meant to have both status and an influence over her. Clara took most of this patiently, but with some reservation. She seemed not to mind or not to show that she minded being reduced through my exploration; however, she also had strong clarity and awareness of her feelings to bring her occasional differentiation and anger.

In contrast, my actual therapist, Lesley, minded being objectified. She was challengingly puzzled as to why I would have spent most of the time in the session trying to seduce her and to create an eroticised atmosphere in which most of the discussion and bodily reactions had an erotic undertone. As an outcome of these clashes, I talked about my grandmother Julia, who daydreamed with me that we would live together in a white house and get married; then I explored the different types of masculinity that were available in my life. There were two men that influenced me a lot as a child, and they could not have been more different: my father and *wujek* Janek ("*wujek*" means uncle).

My father was a gentleman and an intellectual. He always carried two handkerchiefs, one for himself and another for women. He had never spoken overtly about sexuality but sometimes he liked to make a joke with an erotic undertone that showed his interest in "profanum", and his jovial openness towards sex, masturbation, and homosexuality. At the same time, even in my childhood, I was aware that I had never seen my parents physically and erotically close. As a child, I often made sexual jokes and masturbated even a few times a day. Was that a reaction to the repression of sexuality in my home? How much did the avoidance of the subject have an impact on a child?

The second masculine role model was *wujek* Janek, my mother's brother, a local playboy. His bedroom consisted of a king-size bed, large TV screen, and a German porn calendar on the wall, while a light switch in the lounge was a figure of an erect penis. It was not only that I could find porn videotapes in his house, but also that they were actually mixed with tapes of cartoons on the same shelf, both a rare, exotic, and attractive find for a boy who grew up under communism. I remember the familiar sexual confusion, uncontrollable sweaty excitement watching them or waiting for *wujek* Janek to leave home. He was also surrounded by attractive young women. They also loved the little boy that I was, and so I felt very special in an environment of these attractive women, but also confused due to the sexual undercurrent of my uncle and his friends' behaviour.

For many years, *wujek* Janek was the man that I wanted to be. He had a nice house, large TV, Western clothes and cars, including a Porsche that in post-communist Poland made my friends gather around it in admiration. My father was not attractive for me as a boy: he was not athletic and did not have any desirable attributes for my male friends. The fact that the only books *wujek* Janek possessed on his shelf were written by my father could not possibly have any influence on my viewpoint as a child. At that time, I thought that *wujek* Janek was very much how a man should be and how I would like to be as a man.

In my therapy, I started to discover my father's values and re-evaluate him from a different masculine perspective: his openness towards the world and wisdom that he gained bridging two cultures (post-war German and Polish).

I started to change my approach to women and learned how to be in a long-lasting relationship.

Interestingly, when I wanted to talk about sex and my penis, my therapist used to raise her eyebrows and say with an encouraging smile that it was clear I was Continental. She disclosed that none of her English male clients would ever speak about their genitals that openly. Although we attended to many sexual themes, I felt that it was not a place for talking about sex as a physical act. Sex and genitals were treated metaphorically. For example, sex was a way of achieving other, non-sexual relational needs, or the penis was associated with power. Although these insights were extremely precious and needed at that time of my life, sex was no longer a physical act of bodies, sweat, and sperm. The physicality of this act was removed, and my therapist and I did not have a discussion on the reasons why. Perhaps it was her different approach to intimacy, the need to keep some private things away from exposure, or was she possibly reacting to the widespread fear of litigation and psychotherapeutic ethical codes that are becoming more pre-scriptive and restrictive?

3.2.2 Masculinities in dialogue

Samuels (2016), a psychotherapist and researcher, says that men are trying to seduce female therapists usually, not because of some unconscious dynamics, but simply because they do not know what else to do. The reductionist image of women presented in the culture I was brought up in, transgenerational transition of hegemonic masculinity (see Section 3.2.3), and a learned sense of privilege in my childhood were reasons why it was difficult for me to develop other types of relationship with women.

However, reducing the sexualisation of women to the lack of psychosocial skills amongst men misses the point of what men gain through reduction and objectivisation of women. Bringing my attraction, on a regular basis, to the prac-tice sessions with Clara was an attempt to gain control over the session. When sexuality was brought up, I felt more familiar and at ease being able to avoid the intimacy that I feared, while the power I acquired came through reminding her that her skills are as important or even less important than the way she looks. Interestingly Lesley, the more experienced therapist I was seeing at that time, was openly angered by my way of sexualising her. She had an allergic reaction and brought it to my awareness several times until I could see how I tried to manipulate our relational dynamic in a familiar way. Working with Lesley was a real eye-opener for me and an experience that started the never-ending process of gender reconfiguration. The changes did not happen immediately, but since that time I started to give voice to other masculinities inside me that take the power from the seductive, lonely, and fearful masculinity that I frequently embodied at that time.

Throughout the therapy with Lesley and beyond, I enacted additional masculinities that would stand in a dialogic way with other masculine selves that I had already embodied. The post-structuralist idea of masculinities remaining in contradiction with each other (Haywood and Mac an Ghaill, 2003) seems similar to the gestalt therapy theory view of multiple selves within us that struggle for power (Polster, 1995). Both theories agree that we have many selves that can have multiple representations leading to contradictory behaviours. The integration that gestalt therapy offers is not defined in monistic terms, but in a dynamic, pluralistic figure that is choicefully negotiated in changing field conditions.

> By helping men to examine and experience both the limitations and the benefits of their traditionally masculine tendencies, counsellors can facilitate the integration of various parts of the self. A holistic, integrated man will have choice.
>
> (Novack, Park and Friedman, 2013, p. 487)

That choice, however, is always field dependent (Parlett, 1991). In line with Butler's idea of performativity (2011) that accentuates how we reinforce gender roles through performing gender-related activities, the more I explore new masculinities, the more fluidity and ease I have in embodying them. However, I am aware that older parts of myself can be activated when context enhances a former pattern of performativity. Butler (2011), as does gestalt therapy (Perls, Hefferline and Goodman, 2003), sees individuals as context-dependent and free at the same time.

As I explore earlier in Chapter 2, it is the dialogue that heals and changes the dynamics of power. Being a man means being born into a privileged position that needs to be recognised and questioned. This can only be done in dialogue – this includes not only dialogue across gender, but also men's performative engagement in finding and developing new masculine identities.

What we need in psychotherapy is to increase the diversity of gender performativity. Fragmentation of genders (including masculinities or femininities) will provide an opportunity for internal dialogue and reflections, as well as departures from the old type of hegemonic masculinity that is shaping the field and reconfirming old stereotypes: "Male heterosexuality is so far from monolithic, is in fact manifold and surprising" (Grossmark, 2009, p. 87). This understanding is particularly important for psychotherapy, which started at the end of the 19th century as a healing treatment for women, performed by men (Samuels, 2016). Consideration must be given to men's motivation in becoming psychotherapists in terms of the gender dynamics mentioned earlier (Ibidem, 2016) and to how psychotherapy can address these inequalities. More diversifications of my male identities come with further exploration of the history of masculinity in my family.

3.2.3 Transgenerational transition of masculinity

When analysed in the context of communism, it is easy to see how different *wujek* Janek and my father were. Both imprisoned under communism, my father for political activity, *wujek* Janek for illegal trading of currency, they ended up with very different attitudes, strengths, and weaknesses. My father seemed broken and depressed, sad in his soul, but also extremely ethical and trustworthy; *wujek* Janek was more determined, focused, and hedonistic; but they also had very different life histories.

Wujek Janek was born in a family that settled in Poland around 150 years ago. They belonged to Vlachs, a Romanian nomadic tribe of mainly shepherds. His parents (my grandparents) ran a pub in the centre of town before communism confiscated all privately owned establishments. They also lost a huge amount of money, as in the 1950s all their savings were invalidated. I guess he had many reasons to live "carpe diem".

My father (see Figure 3.6) was born in 1933 in a German family in an area that currently belongs to Poland called Masuria (Mazury in Polish and Masuren in German) that at the time, and for hundreds of years before, belonged to Germany and formerly to Prussia. His father was a violinist and teacher, and I have no data on his involvement with Nazis. What I am aware of is that my father had a strong fear when I was boyish and angry; he told me that this is something that I must avoid and looked physically afraid and avoidant of any situation like this. The year my father was born Hitler was voted into power, and at that time the deeply impoverished Eastern Prussia (Masurenland) offered him 80% of support. Hitler supported this region afterwards. In 1944, Mazury was the first land "liberated" by the Red Army. They were extremely cruel and took a revenge on local Germans, which included sexual violence.

My father would never speak about this time, but Aleksandr Solzhenitsyn portrayed it in his poem written in Eastern Prussia:

> It's not been burned, just looted, rifled.
> A moaning by the walls, half muffled:
> the mother's wounded, half alive.
> The little daughter on the mattress,
> Dead. How many have been on it?
> A platoon, a company perhaps?
> A girl's been turned into a woman,
> a woman turned into a corpse.
> The mother begs, "Soldier, kill me!"
> (Solzhenitsyn, 1977, p. 41)

My paternal grandfather spent over a year in prison while other parts of the family were deported to Germany. I do not know what happened at that time when my father was 11, but I am aware that he was never able to watch a rape scene on TV and always had to leave the living room. The family was forced to change their name from Küntzel to Kincel. My father changed his Polish schools

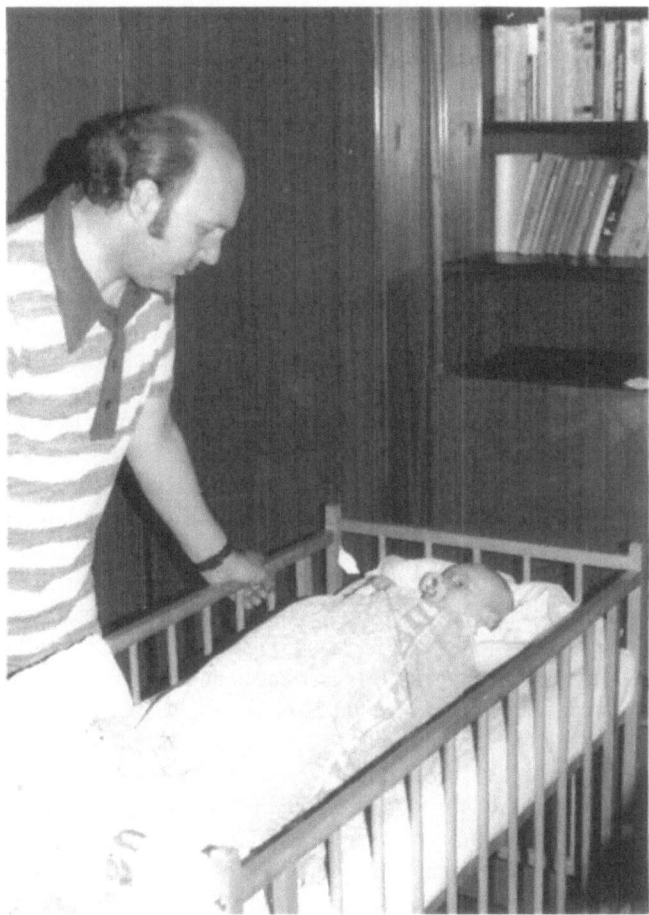

Figure 3.6 Summer 1980 – the gaze exchange between my father and me
Source: Personal photograph.

11 times due to his misbehaviour which, I believe, was associated with bullying and his learning to speak Polish.

After the death of Stalin in 1956, there was a wave of changes amongst all communist countries, and my father eagerly worked to make them happen. When, in 1957, it was obvious that these changes would not be implemented, my father took part in a strike and was one of the 530 arrested at that time and subsequently spent a year in a political labour prison. He left this prison with a ban from attending all universities for the next five years, and with tuberculosis, which cost him a lung. After completing his degree, he was sent by the government to work as a schoolteacher on the top of a mountain in Southern Poland where he had eight students, in six different year groups, and about three hours of hiking to the nearest town. His career as a historian was highly censored, and so he started to study the mountains where he was sent, focusing on the history of tourism and local towns. Most probably, it was the time when he started to overuse alcohol, a habit that stayed with him until his last days.

My fear of my sexual power and penetration has a wider socio-political context, and my father's fear of masculine power and sense of being disempowered by the various institutions must have played a major role in this. In therapy, I was discovering how I often speak with a muted voice, being afraid of appearing too dominant or loud. I experimented with undoing my gentle slouch and looking up rather than down. The bullying that I experienced on my estate seemed like a recreation of my father's story, with aggressive boys I had to hide from and my sense of being different for speaking a different dialect.

Research studies locate transgenerational trauma within epigenetic coding (Yehuda and Bierer, 2009; Yehuda et al., 2016). Some of the studies in epigenetics focus on the transgenerational transmission of stress (Rodgers et al., 2015) and early trauma (Gapp et al., 2014) through sperm. They claim that microRNA enzymes are responsible for transmitting stress to future generations, which can last even a couple of generations. These studies focus on men, but there is a correlation between women's early life experiences and stress during pregnancy on their infant's mental health (Gray et al., 2017).

Coming from the phenomenological perspective, I do not contest the research listed earlier, but my focus both as a researcher and psychotherapist is on how these traumas were passed through embodied practices and experiences.

Ruppert (2008) defines his transgenerational way of working as an integration of trauma and attachment theory, and describes how, through day-to-day activities, trauma is passed on to babies and children, who learn the world from their parents. In Chapter 2, I illustrated how my prejudices towards Polish people were an effect of observing my father and introjecting his way of viewing the world. In the introduction to this chapter, I give an example of embodying my father's trauma of communism. I remember learning from him how to breathe, being next to him. Having only one lung after the tuberculosis in his 20s, he had a distinct way of breathing that I found myself repeating in my adult life as if I too only had one lung. Body posture, body structure, way of breathing, blood pressure and heartbeat, indeed the body is a product of context, as Butler (1993) reminds us.

In the context of my childhood when I was bullied by other boys, I turned towards the masculinity that *wujek* Janek presented, hiding my father's teaching deeply inside. Referring to a period of my life when I focused on my career and earning money while neglecting my family, my sister challenges me in this interview:

AK: I wanted to be like *wujek* Janek. I thought I will be better that way; then the material things took over, I felt better as I owned more.

MY SISTER: **Aha, and why did you not like what our father presented? I liked him fully. I was against everything that they [Uncle Janek and his brother] present and I was with our father.**

AK: Yeah.

MY SISTER: **Why did you like them, but not our father? Do you know what is going on here?**

AK: They were closer to me than our father. Uncle spent more time with me.

MY SISTER: **So, dad was further away?**

AK: Yes.

MY SISTER: **He didn't spend time with you at that time?**

AK: First, he did not spend much time with me, but second, Janek was somebody that was liked on our estate, while they made jokes about our father . . .

MY SISTER: **Aha.**

AK: When Janek visited everyone was asking, what car is this? And our father could not even drive.

MY SISTER: **So, he wasn't a male role model for you?**

AK: No.

MY SISTER: **And he was for me.**

AK: He is now for me, too.

This part of the interview shows how my masculinity was negotiated from early childhood. How my father's traumatised experience of masculinity resulted in him being more detached from me and the boyishness that I needed to experiment with. When I was a victim of harassment and bullying, my father did not protect me, which partly resulted in my early rejection of him and the masculinity he presented. Although I embraced *wujek* Janek's masculinity, I could not sustain it in my adult life where I needed more mature masculinities, especially in relation to women.

The two father figures I had looked very polarised, almost grotesque characters: a cliché of a sensitive man who struggles with the world and a playboy. As shown in Chapter 2, collective gestalts have a dialectic nature that is performed often through a conflict of two polar, even slightly grotesque, characters. What we study here is not the real characters of my ancestors, but my perception of them, my recreation of their characters through this text that was motivated by my situation and ideas about masculinity at the time of writing. Thus, this text is an attempt to work with the collective gestalt by giving voice to both sides and beginning to analyse the cultures that produced this split. Beyond the impact of my family history, there is also the national history and national trauma that became sedimented in the form of the split between victims, perpetrators, and rescuers.

To study psychological trauma is to come face to face both with human vulnerability in the natural world and with the capacity for evil in human nature.

> To study psychological trauma means bearing witness to horrible events. When the events are natural disasters or "acts of God," those who bear witness sympathize readily with the victim. But when the traumatic events are of human design, those who bear witness are caught in the conflict between victim and perpetrator. It is morally impossible to remain neutral in this conflict. The bystander is forced to take sides.
>
> (Herman, 2015, pp. 7–8)

Both my father and I oscillate between the various parts of the so-called drama triangle of victim, perpetrator, and rescuer (Karpman, 1968) that has both a personal and collective dimension. Herman (2015) makes a direct link between experiencing societal trauma and embodying these positions. The victim part of me referred to being bullied and choosing people in my life who disrespected my boundaries. The rescuer was inherited from my father's need to take care of others, especially women, and later choosing a helping profession. Perhaps even this piece of research is motivated by my need to rescue through promoting dialogue and directing attention to the wider collective background. The perpetrator can be seen in this text in the way I objectivise women, but it is also connected with the rebellious spirit of men in my family or anger at my mother for not meeting my needs (see Section 3.3.4). The challenge I received from my therapist Lesley and the constant sense of emptiness that I felt in the embodiment of hegemonic masculinity led me to re-evaluate my relationship with women, and today my sessions with Clara would look very different. At the same time, the pull to join the drama triangle positions of victim, perpetrator, and rescuer is very strong, including my private life and culture.

The drama triangle dynamic had an impact on the mentality of Polish men who feel collectively victimised. This dynamic of victim-perpetrator is illustrated by Datta, who undertook visual narrative research of 20 Polish men working on construction sites in the UK between 2005 and 2006:

> The visual narratives of the Polish participants suggest complex constructions of gender identities and masculinities that make references to a socialist past where the struggles of men to "survive" are seen as justifications of crude humour around sexual violence. These struggles construct ideas of a heterosexual masculinity that does not necessarily regard women as objects of sexual violence, but rather men as the "victims" of a socialist state.
>
> (2009, p. 207)

Although the current conservative Polish government of the Law and Justice party conducts discussions on the inferiority of women towards men, the attitude of ignoring and perpetrating sexual violence and gender inequality in Poland spreads beyond the voters of the conservative government. My findings and Datta's research (2009) suggest that the victimisation of Polish men is both a cause and justification for some of these inequalities, and that violence started before the socialist regime – during the Second World War or even before. Poland has been under a partition that can be compared to colonisation between the Austro-Hungarian Empire, Russia, and Germany for almost 200 years before the First World War. Polish people suffered a sense of humiliation of not being able to have their own country or even schooling in Polish, and the threat of annihilation if they rebelled. The myth of Polish survival is linked to both Polish victimisation as well as rebellion which, in all cases, ended with severe consequences.

Throughout his life my father seemed to be a rebel who was punished by imprisonment and suspension at his university; thus, am I rebellious in a similar Polish way, using the autoethnographic methodology and writing about my sexuality? Am I trying to recreate a similar dynamic of questioning the societal, academic, and psychotherapeutic status quo and what are the implications (see more in Section 7.4.1)? Researching sexuality, Irvine concludes that "sexuality researchers have attempted for over a century to establish academic legitimacy in the face of deep cultural anxieties about their subject of study" (2014, p. 633); so, yet again, I am choosing a difficult path that creates tension and possible dramatic events that are often recreated by traumatised people and explained through the drama triangle (Karpman, 1968). Or am I compensating for the repression of the sexual field both in my family and the Catholic society I was brought up in?

3.2.4 Sexualised field

Although the relational psychotherapy literature usually describes relationships between two people, I am also interested in how certain feelings affect wider networks: field (Lewin, 1952), situation (Staemmler, 2010; Wollants, 2012), or atmosphere (Francesetti, 2015). It is sometimes possible to experience going to a new place with great music and an atmosphere that makes us slightly more flirtatious than usual or where we find ourselves smiling more than usual. These are moments when we become aware of the erotic field (Clemmens, 2010), which is an important and powerful field operating around and within us. When describing my childhood, I suggested that the lack of intimacy between my parents affected me as a child in a way that I felt much of their sexual tension. My father's negative response towards my boyishness, embedded in his war trauma fear of sexual violence intensified my need to keep my sexual energy retroflected (held back). On top of that was the Catholic Church with its requirement of regular confessions of even erotic thoughts. I was not supported to develop healthy mechanisms to deal with my sexuality, and this led to a lot of anxiety that often led to a type of objectivisation called sexualisation. My frequent need to sexualise was directly related to the lack of permission to discuss sexuality as prohibited by the Catholic Church, my father's trauma, and my parents' avoidance of this subject. Furthermore, the peer pressure on embodying heteronormativity (see Chapter 4) and sexualising women and relationships with women added to the sexualisation it co-created.

My concern is that the current attitude to sex in psychotherapy is similar to the situation in my family home and may lead to sexualisation or a denial of sexuality that, in consequence, can lead to sexual abuse, as has happened in a number of religious organisations that do not address or permit sexuality (Spraitz and Bowen, 2016). The mildest form of the retroflected sexual field in psychotherapy may manifest in neglect or avoidance of certain topics.

Contemporary psychotherapists contribute to the creation of the repressed sexualised field by avoiding the erotic field. For different reasons it is a difficult decision whether to move attention to the erotic field in therapy for male, female, and non-binary therapists. Yet, it is important that we build supportive relationships with our clients in which we can talk about sexuality, with all the baggage it brings, ranging from unfulfilled needs to powerful work on the abuse some of our clients have experienced.

> I now understand that courage in therapy is also the courage for the patient and the therapist each to claim her/his own authentic experience of self. In this the therapist must lead the way. [. . .] I believe in intersubjective cocreation of therapeutic reality, but I also believe in a differential responsibility for the therapeutic outcome. If our patients could create a path out of their problems on their own initiative, they would not need us.
>
> (Hyde, 2006, p. 70)

Writing about sexuality in psychotherapy, Hyde (2006) accentuates his own authentic experiences. Above everything, our sexuality and sexual resonance is the main indicator of what is present in our relationships with clients, and a prolonged lack of it is a worrying sign of prejudices or repression (see Chapter 4).

There is a major cultural difference between my treatments in Poland and England when it comes to sexuality. In my therapy in England, sex was a metaphor for wider societal or interpersonal difficulties, words describing the sexual act and organs were usually not used unless I brought them up. Although in Victorian times sexuality was broadly discussed and terms such as lesbian, heterosexual, nymphomaniac, or orgasm were commonly used (Furneaux, 2014), it did not strongly impact on behaviour. The term "Victorian sexuality" describes British reservations around sexuality which includes deep societal shame at the prospect of being driven by anything other than rational thinking. Free expression of emotions and affections was not permitted, while self-control to restrain feeling and affection is a virtue. Figure 3.7 shows the kind of advice given by my autocorrector that is most probably based on my use of language, but it is a warning that many academics researching sexuality hear (Irvine, 2014). Neoliberalism enhances what Irvine (2014) calls *speaker burden,* which he uses to describe the discrimination and shame that awaits sex researchers. Both in psychotherapy and academia there is the ever-present fear of litigation and accusation of sexual misconduct. There seems to be an association between touch and abuse, as if sexual abuse could not happen without touch and that all touch is inherently sexually and

> ☒
>
> ## Possibly confused word: erection
>
> ### Did you mean: election?
>
> The word **erection** doesn't seem to fit this context. Consider replacing it with a different one.

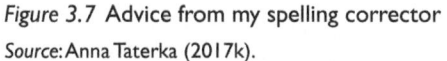

Figure 3.7 Advice from my spelling corrector
Source: Anna Taterka (2017k).

abusive. It seems that in this culture, we are constantly obsessed with sex, making rules that regulate our life to avoid any possible eroticism, when simultaneously our sexual awareness, knowledge of our sexual needs, and ways to express them as well as the ability to notice subtle sexual power dynamics are prohibited. This creates a scary image of culture obsessed with prohibition that leads to lack of awareness and abuse.

When experiencing therapy in Poland, it was possible to speak about sex in an open way; the atmosphere was both tense and full of assurance that it was okay to talk about sex. There is a resemblance to confession in mainly Catholic Poland where, as a child, I was invited to describe my sexual experiences, be it a fantasy or masturbation. Of course, after confessional disclosures I was expecting a judgement, and so Polish psychotherapists make an enormous effort to show that they listen without judgement. There seems to be a split in Polish society that is clearly manifested in politics, on the use of contraception, abortion, LGBTQI rights, and sexual freedom, between conservative Catholic beliefs and the liberal attitude of assurances described earlier (more about this in Chapter 4). Although the conservative government is not usually supported by psychotherapists, the conservative ideas and sexual repressions have a profound effect on the trainee therapists that I teach in Poland. The tension and anger in the LBGTQI+ psycho-therapists are much greater than in England. They live in fear, carefully choosing places where they can come out as an attack could be both physical as well as political. Being gay is mentioned as the main reason for social isolation in Poland (Hearn and Pringle, 2006, p. 138) and it is estimated that 30% of young Polish LGBTQI+ people attempt suicide (Zeeman et al., 2017, p. 215). In one of the groups I facilitated in Poland, I invited the whole training group to walk around the room, embodying a person who did not identify with any of the genders, and this brought a strong depressive feeling to the group. Whether these are possible real feelings of the androgynous people in Poland or a projection of the trainee therapists in the room, it presents a strong image of discomfort regarding non-traditional embodiment of genders. More discussion on this subject is presented in Section 4.1.4.

It seems that the conflict between attitudes towards sexuality is much more open and hurtful in Poland, while in England it is hidden and regulated. In both places there seems to be a struggle between allowance and prohibition. In this chapter, the themes of erection as cultural and transgenerational are interwoven with its biological and relational meanings. My focus on sexuality is influenced by my British therapist as I am interested in the lived, sensuous body as a product of culture. Next, I return to the micro level, analysing how I react bodily to falling in love.

3.3 Sexuality negotiated relationally

Collective factors mediate the collective gestalt of masculinity through medicalisation, class, social system, and the way people are treated in society because of their gender. I illustrated that although alternative approaches to medicine can offer a more holistic view of the person, the diagnosis and treatment can be reductionist, reinforcing old stereotypes. The example of falling in love is used to evidence how the embodiment of a collective gestalt of masculinity is a function of culture, relational dynamics, and the support available in our life.

3.3.1 Autoethnography: falling in love

A few years after my therapy with Lesley, I fell in love. At that time, I did not bring it to my therapist, but I was seeing a Traditional Chinese Medicine (TCM) practitioner who, after checking my pulse, asked me what difficulty I was experiencing. I asked him for clarification, and he said that my yang (masculine energy) was totally depleted and through my pulse, he diagnosed a large quantity of shame and fear; he even asked me if I had problems with erection. I sat more deeply in my chair, took a breath, and admitted that I had fallen in love. That TCM practitioner had known me for over a year back then and was surprised to see such abnormality in my system. I was embarrassed to be seen so much through my bodily reactions. His feedback helped me to realise how little confidence I had and how I downgraded myself in idealising the person I met. It seemed that my anxiety about whether I would be liked the way I am had moved me to a state where I started doing many things for the other person that included glorifying them. At first, I started to trust that my partner wanted to be with me and like me. As basic as it sounds, it is a necessary invitation for me to feel sexual. At the same time, the male practitioner prescribed me herbs that could help me to feel stronger.

3.3.2 Masculine medicine and psychotherapy

The split between pathological and normal was one of the most difficult dichotomies I had to overcome when discovering my masculinity. On the one hand, there is a medical and deeply entrenched cultural model that looks for normality and faults in people. In this model, I am a man who could be diagnosed as suffering from sexual dysfunction or inhibition at certain times. The complexity of the body is being reduced here to an organ (Deleuze and Guattari, 1987; Fox, 2012). Second is an acceptance model, in which I treat myself as someone who is healthy and in tune with his body. Body is seen as an assemblage that is affecting and is affected at the same time (Fox, 2012; Fox and Alldred, 2017). If at the beginning of a relationship I feel rather understandable anxiety and fear, would it truly be a sign of health to desensitise (switch off or mute bodily sensations) in that moment and make love?

The current ideology of masculine performance (Bordo, 2000; Orbach, 2010) is based on desensitisation and sexual achievements, and although men are often accused of not feeling much, we are also socialised to take these roles. Recent analysis on how Viagra is advertised shows that "performance" is the keyword (Orbach, 2010) and in some of the West, Viagra medication is subsidised by the government, for example, the US Army spent $41 million on the blue pill in 2016 (Eustachewich, 2017). Although I understand that loss of erection can be a problematic issue, offering medication on a massive scale deflects from many relational difficulties, fear of ageing, and issues related to masculinity that psychotherapy, couples therapy, and alternative approaches to medicine can help to address. It seems that government and medicine support men's silencing of emotions and relational difficulties (Real, 1999).

Furthermore, the blue pill is labelled as a solution not only for erection, but also for depression (see Figure 3.8). "We exist at a particular historical moment in a society that promotes at least two versions of 'the blues', discontent, and pills, specifically those pills modeled after the original 'little blue pill', Viagra" (Loe, 2006, p. 22). This association is reinforced by scientific research claiming that the use of Viagra increases the wellbeing of men (Montorsi, Padma-Nathan and Glina, 2006), when ignoring the fact that the wellbeing of men in the first place has a strong impact on erection. Serotonin and dopamine, hormones that affect and regulate our wellbeing and sense of happiness, play an important role in creating erection and ejaculation (Giuliano, 2011). However, patients claim that long-term use of antidepressants that aim to regulate these hormones causes not only a deflated feeling, but also the loss of erection (Edemariam, 2017). Although sexual

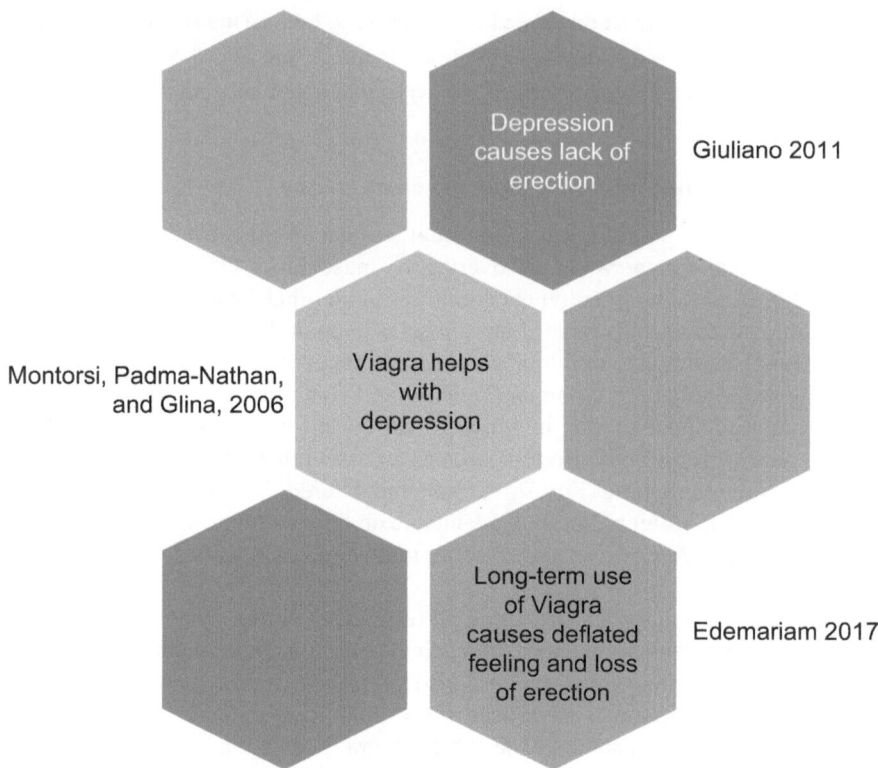

Figure 3.8 Paradoxes of prescribing Viagra for depression

satisfaction brings positive feelings to life, there is a concern about studies that associate penile hardness with life satisfaction. Interviewing men of different ages using Viagra, Loe (2006, p. 32), notices:

> According to these men, Viagra can be seen as a treatment for lost, "diminished", troubled, or incomplete masculinity. And masculinity, in their words, means youth, virility, confidence, size, substance, and general sense of worth.

There seems to be little or no insight amongst these men about alternative forms of attending to ageing, confidence, and self-worth. They seem to be locked in the hegemonic type of masculinity that is based on potency. It reduces men's anxiety by allowing them to be predictable and consistent (Loe, 2006, p. 37) but, in fact, taking Viagra does not reduce the anxiety but adds another anxiety of whether men would ever be able to make love without medication (Fox and Alldred, 2017, p. 123). Although psychotherapy opens masculinity to other dimensions that include the acceptance of anxiety and uncertainty, it may also be promoting a masculinity that is fixed and prescribed.

A key book on masculinity for psychotherapists (currently mandatory reading for students in a training institute where I work), entitled *Iron John* (Bly, 2013), seems to both promote and dismantle stereotypes about men and masculinity. Bly "resonate[s] with the fashionable angst of the new man, while simultaneously celebrating a version of macho masculinity" (Haywood and Mac an Ghaill, 2003, p. 28). Although, according to Bly (2013), women can be strong and men can have emotions, the goal of the man is to find his inner "warrior" and "hairy man". This traditional view of masculinity is popular amongst psychotherapists who encourage their clients to return to a traditional masculinity rather than to question masculinities and invent new ones. Suggesting fixed ideas about gender can be as abusive as conversion pseudotherapy (see Chapter 4), where health is associated with only one sexual orientation. Suggesting to clients that they need to return to traditional sexuality could be a way of avoiding, by some psychotherapists, discussions on gender within the therapeutic context. A similarly damaging view could be to believe that men need to have strong erections when required to feel happy. My first therapist, and later Clara, accepted my need to exercise strong and sexualised masculinity, while Lesley engaged in an argument with me each time I attempted to objectify her.

I think that addressing gender in therapy is almost as difficult as addressing sexuality. The inevitable amount of anger, but also shame and guilt, it may create seem to be good enough reasons to look for a safe escape into gender stereotyped roles.

"Erectile difficulties are real. But so are the fears that men have about such difficulties, as well as cultural ideals conflating potency, manhood, and individualism" (Loe, 2006, p. 44). Later in this chapter, I move on to describe how the embodiment of culturally mediated collective gestalts are negotiated relationally through our enduring relational themes (Jacobs, 2017) and current situation (Wollants, 2012).

3.3.3 Sexuality as a relational phenomenon

The relational turn in psychotherapy (Benjamin, 2018; Frie and Orange, 2013) contributed to seeing most psychological issues as relational phenomena. In the literature, there seems to be a double understanding of relational sexuality, as some writers use this term to talk about sexuality within a relationship as opposed to casual sex with strangers (Talmadge and Talmadge, 1986). By relational sexuality, I mean the inevitable dependency of sexual behaviours and feelings on relational and emotional dynamics. Furthermore, I suggest that our sexuality depends not only on the relationship with a partner, but also on our experiences in our families, social, and cultural dynamics.

Various aspects of our sexuality are dependent on the relationship, be it a low sexual drive (Talmadge and Talmadge, 1986), sexual frequency and satisfaction, and types of sexual activity and the use of contraceptives (Willetts, Sprecher and

Beck, 2004, p. 59), but it is important to recognise the impact of traditional, hegemonic masculine research that locates men's sexual inhibitions in the arena of
mainly biological dysfunctions.

A current quantitative study of erectile dysfunction demonstrated the existence
of intrapsychic, relational, and organic components of both achieving and maintaining erections (Corona et al., 2005). They noticed that patients who have difficulty in maintaining an erection do not usually suffer from organic conditions,
but are affected by intrapsychic and relational factors (2005, p. 256). According
to Corona et al. (2005), patients who have difficulty in achieving an erection are
usually experiencing an organic condition and they also seem to have much higher
anxiety scores than men who are able to achieve, but unable to maintain, an erection. Further research is needed to examine the impact of stress and anxiety on their
physical wellbeing and, subsequently, achievement of an erection. Nevertheless,
the research mentioned earlier should alert therapists to use different approaches
with male clients with difficulty maintaining or achieving erection. Although during my first therapy I reported to my therapist that I was able to achieve an erection, I was still invited to practise some bioenergetic exercises to stimulate energy
in my lower back. That was not the treatment I needed at that time.

While medical studies link relaxation (Corona et al., 2005) and happiness (Giuliano,
2011) with an erection, contemporary gestalt literature positions relaxation and happiness within the relational matrix (Frank, 2001; Hycner and Jacobs, 1995; Yontef,
2009). Although relaxation is usually seen as an embodied individual process, the
ability to "yield with" (Frank and Barre, 2011) and "trust the yield" depends on the
safety we experience and experienced within the matrix of relationships.

> From a field theoretical gestalt perspective, sexual difficulties are relational,
> even if only one of the partners subjectively feels sexually unsatisfied, inad-
> equate, unable to experience pleasure, unaware of his or her own needs, con-
> fused regarding his or her choice of partners, or anxious or depressed in the
> course of coming to terms with his or her sexual orientation.
>
> (Amendt-Lyon, 2013, p. 571)

Our sexuality is not just an individual phenomenon, but an outcome of attach-
ments we have and have had in our life (Stephan and Bachman, 1999), as well as
the wider socio-political field.

3.3.4 Sexuality and attachment

Although all contact including sexual contact needs to be understood in gestalt
therapy as a part of the relational field, each person brings to that field enduring relational themes (Jacobs, 2011). We learn these themes usually early on in
significant relationships; however, they evolve and are created throughout the
life span. Attachment theory has classified some of these relationships (Bowlby,
1997); however, it is important to remember that attachment styles do not depend

only on the individual presenting this style, but also on the quality of the relationship between that person and the situation.

According to attachment theory (Bowlby, 1997), we embody different styles of attachment that can be traced to our childhood. Although I do not introduce his theory here, I want to acknowledge a body of research that studies the relationship between attachment styles and sexuality (for example: Brennan and Shaver, 1995; Simpson, Wilson and Winterheld, 2004; and Stephan and Bachman, 1999). The attachment style that I had at the beginning of my relationship can be described as having large quantities of fear: of abandonment, closeness, and intimacy. The drama of this position lies in the fact that the person both wants to be close, but also fears it greatly. My mother provides a useful insight of my attachment in the first ten minutes of the interview:

> [My mother] I remember your room; you were different from [your sister]; she pulled on everything. I always needed to focus on her, you were different. You went to your room, had your toy cars, here is c-a, c-a [car], you named all your toys. You could sit and play. From time to time you ran to me to tell me something, to lift you, to hold you, cuddle. Once you said that the best times are with mummy. You liked to be cuddled; you were a big darling and I like children like this. Maybe I kiss them too much. Ola [Olga] used to run away from me [when] she had enough. I remember you squatting and playing with your toys; you could organise a lot of things by yourself.

That feedback resonates with my embodied perception of my childhood that oscillates between loneliness and overstimulation by women's needs (see Sections 3.1.1). The loneliness is seen in my mother's praise for my independence from the time I was very young. She suggested that the demands my sister was making were difficult for her to meet and that she felt a relief when I was playing by myself. She does not make a link that perhaps my need for space was related to overstimulation and a lack of awareness of my needs when we were close.

Attachment theory is an attempt to classify intimate behaviours, but as with most theories on human behaviour, it inevitably fails to explain every person's experience with diverse experiences of intimacy and individual histories. What is more certain is that there is a correlation between how we engage or disengage bodily in intimate situations and enduring relational themes. We can gain much information about ourselves and our clients by knowing how they and we engage in sexual and erotic relationships.

Referring to Frank and Barre's theory of six fundamental developmental movements such as yield with, push against, reach for, grasping onto, pull towards, and release from (2011), I see a developmental history in the way we approach sexuality. The traumas either acquired by us or transmitted transgenerationally are felt bodily, and this already affects the way we yield with the significant people in our lives: the vulnerability of reaching out when our lover is next to us and we want to initiate sex; push that is required to get what we want or show what we do not; grasp and pull as a necessary part of seduction, holding or pleasure; as well as a release that is required to orgasm are just some of the movements that we can observe when discussing sexuality. Unfortunately, some therapists use metaphors to deflect from sexuality, rather than using sexuality as a metaphor for other life processes.

Only when I explored my fear related to intimacy in my therapy was I able to understand and feel in tune with my body. My occasional loss of erection was no longer a shameful failure, but a manifestation of relational dynamics and an opening for dialogue. That empathic, caring, and understanding part of me was created and grows to support me, even though sometimes I can still betray it. When falling in love, I completely ignored the relational phenomenon of this state. I took advice and indeed medication from my herbalist to become the stronger man (Section 3.3.1), not paying much attention to what my body was telling me about the speed and perhaps risk of engaging in a relationship. It is a good reminder how even alternative medicine can offer traditionally constructed male roles rather than the acceptance of feelings and the natural pace of building relationships.

3.4 Conclusion

Except for suggestions towards working with sexuality through the paradoxical theory of change (Beisser, 1970), embodied relational attitude, and experimentation, this chapter examines the collective gestalt of my masculinity as an outcome of post-Second World War Poland, communism, post-communism, class, psychotherapy, views on masculinity, and relationships in my life. With such a rich cultural background to study masculinity, this topic has received limited scientific attention in Poland (Hearn and Pringle, 2006), and also in gestalt therapy (Novack, Park and Friedman, 2013). I hope that this chapter encourages dialogue and reflections that provide further insights in the field of masculinity, psychotherapy, and culture.

The change that took place in my therapy has not only impacted the pattern of my sexuality, but it has made a considerable impact on other areas of my life that led to greater acceptance of myself. Furthermore, it allowed me to reduce the shame of feeling that I need to be a man immune to feelings and external influences. I have realised that I am inescapably embedded in the relational and cultural dynamics and my reactions, including sexual reactions, are an outcome of this process.

This chapter illustrates how the free experimenting that touches the boundary of what is appropriate in counselling and psychotherapy is necessary to explore themes that can be easily repressed. Gender studies that include work on masculinity are necessary in the training of psychotherapists to untangle the field that produces bodies that breathe in and out prejudices and repression of uncomfortable themes. The collective gestalts are produced in the meeting between the personal (including early development, life experiences, transgenerational transition of trauma) and the public (including culture, politics, gender). It is this unique association that needs to be examined in relational encounters and which challenges us to look beyond the comfortable. Therapists need to find ways of bringing their own collective wounds and privileges into psychotherapeutic practice, risking a dialogue that may be transformational for both themselves and their clients.

When writing this chapter, I felt a sense of risk. With the current governmental situation in Poland, publishing it would not allow me to find work in public services. Apart from this, there is a risk of losing my reputation as a psychotherapist. Even as a psychotherapist, I associated my success in the field of psychotherapy with my male potency and feared that the disclosure of my occasional impotency will reduce my impact. Having considered these risks by myself and in consultation with my colleagues, I started to wonder how much prejudice there is against showing men's vulnerability. How much of a career is built on the myth of invulnerability? As relational therapists are becoming more vulnerable and open when working with clients, should we not be open for similar exploration in research? Autoethnography allows us to study phenomena at great depth. Having oneself as a research subject, and allowing some years for this exploration, offers unique conditions that have already been used with other sensitive topics (Etherington, 2003). It is the role of autoethnographers to describe but also challenge culture, and to discuss topics that are uncomfortable and important. On a more personal level, I created environments in which my multiple masculinities *intra-act* in a way that do not reinforce the old stereotype of hegemonic masculinity or promote the objectification of women.

There are many different ways masculinity is formed. Earlier in this chapter, I discussed the formation and deconstruction of my sexuality in mainly heterosexual romantic relationships and my transgenerational transition of trauma. However, what is missing here and often in the heteronormative world is the formation of masculinity in relationship between people of the same sex. Anderson (2009) suggests that what he calls *inclusive masculinity* is formed when a spectrum of sexual attraction is allowed in defining masculinity. I will address heteronormative attitudes in the next chapter.

Chapter 4

Embodiment of heteronormativity

Building the field for addressing collective gestalts

4.1 Introduction

Although psychotherapists are keen to discuss sexuality outside of the consulting room, an exploration of Eros proves to be more difficult (Renn, 2013; Cornell, 2003). Some psychotherapists like to call their own sexual reactions towards their clients a countertransference (Hyde, 2006) as this noun provides a way to remove sexual feelings from ourselves. Countertransference means that we are merely reacting to the client's sexuality which we empathically pick up. Even the client's desire towards the therapist is usually called transference, as if two human beings could not be simply attracted to each other. Although relational gestalt therapists believe that feelings in the therapy room are co-created by both the client and the therapist, a discussion about sexual attraction being co-created by both sides rarely occurs (O'Shea, 2000; Cornell, 2003). If sexuality can be a taboo in psychotherapy, discussions on homosexual attraction are permitted even less. Although it is believed that eroticism between same sex therapists and clients occurs regularly, psychotherapists may have difficulty in recognising it (Gabbard, 1996, p. 139). Psychotherapists, as all human beings, are influenced by and dependent on the culture they live in and the norms and prejudices embedded in their culture.

> Therapists are not immune from this. Homophobia is always a block to psychological contact with sexual minority clients regardless of the sexual orientation of the therapist.
>
> (Davies and Aykroyd, 2002, p. 230)

Of course, therapists should keep clear professional boundaries with their clients and not engage in any exploitative activity; however, sexuality is too often labelled as exploitative when it is not. Sensitivity towards a client's sexual and intimate needs depends on how therapists experience their own sexuality, therefore therapists require awareness and maturity regarding their own sexuality and sexual needs.

In this chapter, I will present heteronormativity and fear of sexuality as embodied social processes that serve various purposes in life and in therapy. Through attending to my own examples of embodiments in therapy, heteronormativity will be explored as a field phenomenon (Perls, Hefferline and Goodman, 2003; Parlett,

1991), which includes references to a felt sense of the erotic field. Field theory has been integrated in gestalt therapy from Lewin (1952). Yontef defines field as a "totality of mutually influencing forces that together form a unified interactive whole" (1993, p. 321). Field, also called situation (Wollants, 2012), is both impacting us and is impacted by us, a fluid, constantly changing process. Field is felt through embodiment (Clemmens, 2012), and hence my references to embodied heteronormativity include both reflections on how therapists create heteronormativity as well as how they are affected by it bodily.

Societal prejudices have affected psychotherapy and ethics, and continue to have a negative impact on working with sexuality and touch (except for specific body therapies). Instead of promoting discussion and engagement, which leads to greater awareness of sexual needs and identities, psychotherapy colluded and continues to collude with conservative views, and creates a system in which psychotherapists are often scared of being sued or wrongly accused of sexual misconduct. Some psychotherapeutic misuses and lack of agreed ethical standards in some psychotherapeutic schools (including within gestalt therapy) before the 1980s added to the need for greater control and sensitivity towards abuse in psychotherapeutic practice. However, the sexual secrecy that resulted from it may not only inhibit therapeutic practice, but may also lead to further abuse. This type of therapy is called "safe therapy" as it offers a safer therapy for the therapist, while reducing the impact of the therapy for the client (Samuels, 2003).

Every collective gestalt is silenced by the difficulty of approaching the hate (de Maré, Piper and Thompson, 1991); however, this one has two additional qualities. The first is that the fear of sexuality in the therapy room risks the polarisation into the abuser and abused – doer and done to (Benjamin, 2018) that is the dynamic of power. Second, that masculine identity in our society seems to be particularly challenged by same-sex attraction.

This chapter provides a discussion on therapists' embodied sexual identity. Some consideration will also be given to the heteronormativity present in some psychotherapy trainings, whilst autoethnographic examples will illustrate the therapist's journey, including anonymised descriptions of therapeutic work. Integrating my experiences from British and Polish psychotherapeutic work, I will interweave examples and references from both countries. The term "LGBTQI communities" is used here to cover all people identifying with this term including lesbian, gay, bisexual, trans, queer, and intersex people.

4.1.1 Heteronormativity – personal account

4.1.1.1 2011

> Marek (pseudonym) is a 70-year-old, Polish, jazz double bass player. He said he came to see me for psychotherapy as he was struggling with intimate relationships and did not have a long-standing relationship in his life. It was very clear from the beginning that it would be a therapy full of hope for the future and

grief about an unfulfilled life/about the past. Due to the age gap between us, I realised that I would have to mature quickly to understand his difficulties. Marek mentioned that he was unsure about his sexuality though, at that time, I did not understand that what he meant was that he was sure he was gay. Each week I would see a supervisor to talk about my clients and when I saw my supervisor at the beginning of my work with Marek, my supervisor, a man in his 80s, suggested that Marek's sexual days would be over as at his age sexuality does not play such an important role. This was one of many prejudices I have had to overcome in working with Marek over three years.

Marek was not a person who knew how to speak about his emotions; however, he knew how to tell stories, which were full of wit and intellect. He spoke old Polish without any slang, which I remember hearing in old TV films of the 1950s and I felt very young when, every now and then, I used words such as "cool" or "yeah". At that time, I was balancing my work with Marek between meeting him as he was, and then also inviting him to start noticing and describing his feelings. This was a tricky process as I could see that behind these stories Marek wanted me to see how erudite he was, and my inviting him into this world of feelings and body sensations, a world he had a little knowledge of, would easily trigger fear and shame for him. When he was not reporting much from his internal world, I had plenty of time to explore my own feelings.

Early in the sessions, I was surprised by the experience of hot flushes on my face and warm energy in my pelvis. It was the kind of feeling as if I put my pelvis into a warm bath (before I submerge my whole body), feeling my muscles in this area relax and I could also get a bit light-headed. The feeling was so strong that I knew I could not ignore it when working with him and I spent several sessions thinking about whether I should mention it or not. I was full of embarrassment and realised that my embarrassment was probably mirroring his inhibition to speak about his own feelings and body sensations and that I was, in fact, the one who could stop it. When he came the following week, I disclosed to him my sensations as soon as I started to experience them. At that time Marek's face turned red and he looked at the window. "Is it not obvious that I like you, Adam?" he inquired. At that time, my face became red. It turned out that Marek was worried whether he would be able to work with me as he found me attractive.

4.1.1.2 2009

Two years before seeing Marek, I was in personal therapy with Tom, who was a body therapist from Sweden. I chose him after a few years with a female therapist to focus on my relationships with men. Exploring my relationship with my father, I noticed that what I loved about me and my father were the moments I could lie next to him and hug him. For several sessions, I was lying on Tom's lap and

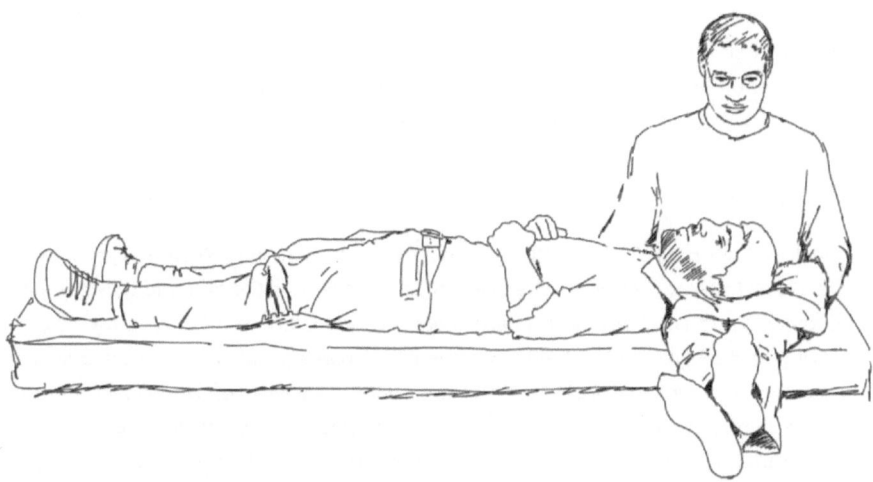

Figure 4.1 On the knees of Tom – a body therapy and heteronormativity
Source: Anna Taterka (2017g).

continuing our discussions (see Figure 4.1). Soon, I started having intrusive thoughts about my attraction to him and his attraction to me. I opened this topic with him, saying how difficult it was for me to be intimate with him and not sexual. I noticed that to feel safe I had to create a boundary between sexuality and intimacy as if they belonged to two distinct categories. It was, in fact, my anxiety which was leading me to compartmentalise. Could I find him attractive and accept his attraction without needing to deny intimacy? Is it okay to fancy my therapist, especially if before I identified myself as straight? Is it okay to fancy my male therapist and lie on his knees?

4.1.1.3 2006

During the first year of my psychotherapy training in England (I had already undertaken almost three years of gestalt training in Poland), I started a student placement and saw my second-ever client for their second session. In this session, the client disclosed to me that he was a gay man. I did what I thought a therapist should do at that moment and asked him how it was for him to share that with me. I asked when he came out, what reactions there had been and whether he was dating someone right now. Interestingly, the client never returned nor let me know that he quit his therapy. At that time, I was working with an analytic supervisor, who was gay, who suggested that the client may have told me he was gay because he fancied me. In my naivety, I replied that I am straight and perhaps I have not picked up on the transference in my body. My supervisor replied,

"Adam, transference works beyond age and gender. You have not picked up this transference because you are homophobic." This was a shock. Although I believe that this statement was a harsh remark to make to a new therapist, it may have been grounded in the supervisor's own anger towards homophobia. I also think it was a correct analysis and the process was named accurately.

4.1.1.4 1997

Andrew (see Figure 4.2) was living with a friend of mine who, when I was an angry teenager, I used to stay with often overnight. Andrew was the first and only gay man I knew in the small southern Polish town where I grew up. He had a mysterious ability to distinguish other hidden gay men in a crowd (a skill which enabled finding partners and avoiding problems in a homophobic society before Grindr), and we often clubbed together with a group of friends. One night we came back to the flat alone after a night of clubbing and ended up sitting on the sofa together, looking at the rising sun. Sipping cocktails and having a nice conversation, I started to feel attracted to him and he looked at me tenderly. At that time, I started to feel a pain in my back and remember pulling my pelvis back, locking energy inside. I think I quickly started speaking about my ex-girlfriend and went to sleep.

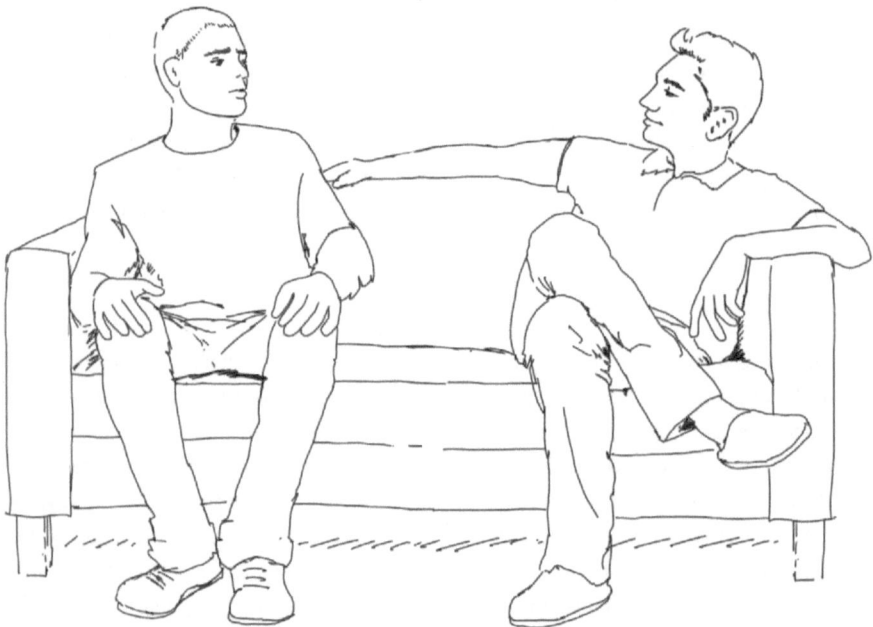

Figure 4.2 Fear of homoeroticism in my teenage years: Andrew and me
Source: Anna Taterka (2017c).

4.1.1.5 1991

My mother was a lawyer for a mining company and, in a communist regime, this meant we received a modern flat on an estate which belonged to a mine. I was the only middle-class child on the estate and spoke with a different accent – other kids spoke Silesian (a mixture of German and Polish). It was a violent estate, but even more violence was going on outside, due to an equivalent of postcode wars in the town in the 1980s. I did not want to fight and even though I attended kung-fu classes, I was defenceless when faced with a street fight. Although initially I felt confident to experiment with various gender expressions (see Figure 4.3), I soon learned that I needed to present myself as a man, and more precisely, as a straight man. Other kids often called me a fag and I found myself a girlfriend rather early both to be seen as straight and to have an excuse to be away from other boys. With this withdrawal, the name "fag" did not disappear, but intensified.

4.1.2 Embodied transference and the erotic field

Transference is a widely used term in psychoanalysis to describe a relationship in which a client reacts towards a therapist as if the therapist were someone else. For example, a client may be afraid that the therapist will be judgemental towards her as her mother had been, and so she keeps herself quiet, transferring her mother's judgemental attitude on to the therapist. Gestalt therapy has adopted transference from psychoanalysis, defining it as a moment when someone reacts according to the old field conditions and is not able to respond to the here-and-now situation (Perls, Hefferline and Goodman, 2003, pp. 221–222). This definition was challenged by the relational movement which claims that even old transferred feelings take place in the current field conditions, which also take an active part in creating these experiences (Jacobs, 2011). Instead of transference, Jacobs, a relational gestalt therapist, proposes the term *enduring relational themes* (2017) to accentuate the dependency of a theme on the relationship within which it occurs. The relational turn brought back the psychotherapist as a real human being, who is constantly impacting upon and impacted by the situation and by other human beings.

Erotic transference is a type of transference which has been widely described amongst various psychotherapeutic schools and theorists. An illustrative book by Hajcak and Garwood (1987) describes 17 ways in which we may use our sexuality to gain results, other than just pleasure. For example, sexuality could be the only acceptable way for an emotionally rigid man to request intimacy from his partner: instead of asking for a cuddle, a stroke, or a kiss, he initiates sex. Similarly, in my psychotherapeutic practice, sexuality can have many meanings. Sometimes it may be less related to a real sexual desire, as when a client needs to feel safe or when the client needs to feel closer to me, or for other reasons which may be related to early life experiences. For some people, however, the feeling of sexual heat is important for purely sexual reasons; they need a supportive space to be aware of their sexuality and of sexual power, permission to be present as a sexual being. For

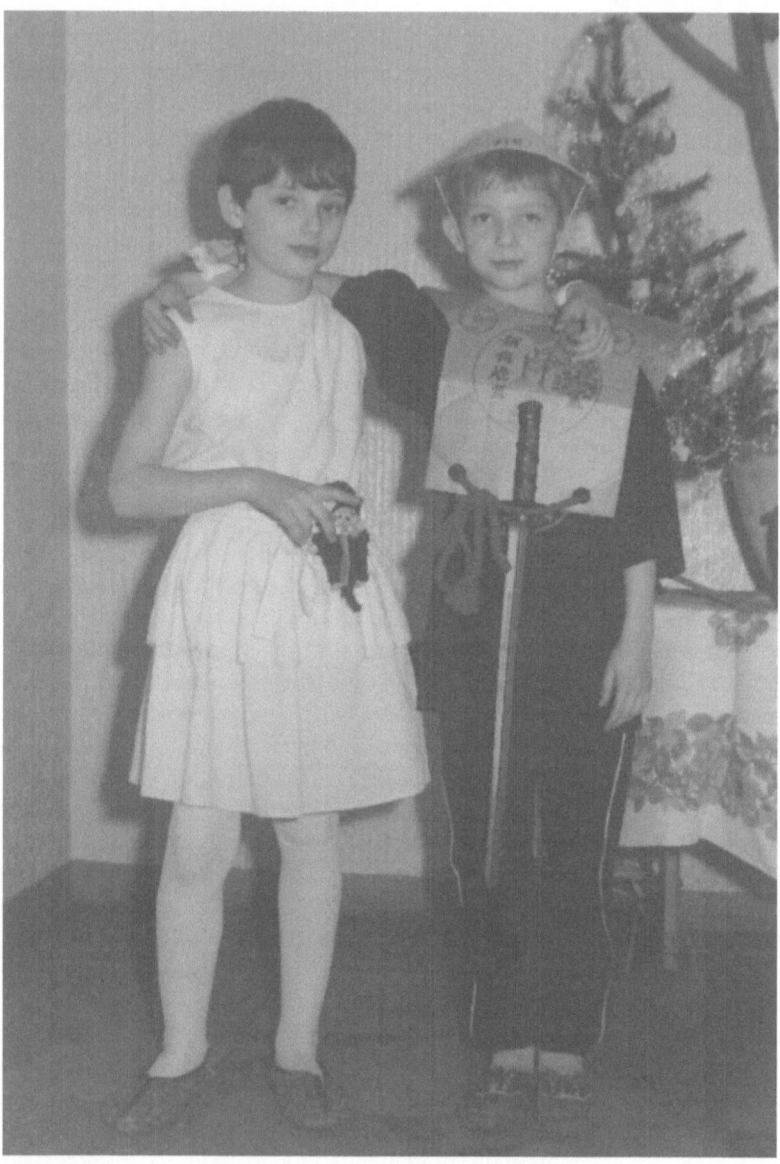

Figure 4.3 1985 – a costume party in my nursery
Source: Personal photograph.

example, as one of my clients was coming out of her depression, she realised her libido was coming back. Contemporary psychoanalysis which, similar to gestalt, includes both relational and individualistic paradigms, does not exclude either the reality or transference of love:

[T]he patient's love is both real, in terms of a unique current relationship, and unreal, in that it has elements of past internalized object relations that are reactivated in the therapeutic dyad.

(Renn, 2013, p. 141)

Since sexuality and eroticism fulfil so many roles, attention to sexuality and sexual energy is necessary in the consulting room (Samuels, 2003). In line with the belief that a therapist's anxiety is a major block to erotic transference in therapy (Gabbard, 1996; Samuels, 2003), I believe that therapists need support to feel comfortable with their own sexual energy to attend to their clients' sexuality. The sense of warmth moving down my pelvis (in Section 4.1.1.1) is just an example of how sexuality can be embodied; each person has a unique way of embodying sexual interest or excitement depending on the time, relationship, and context.

An enduring relational theme in gestalt therapy is embodied and can be sensed through an embodied resonance (Frank, 2001). An embodied resonance is a sophisticated, but intuitive process. According to Clemmens (2012), it starts with a great awareness of one's embodiment and of bodily sensations. Breathing and grounding exercises may foster an awareness of our body sensations. Another way to do it is to move awareness through different parts of our bodies, a so-called body scan. The second step is to be able to sense the field outside, in other words, to minimise our attention to our own internally generated sensations as much as possible and to notice, through our bodies, what is happening outside. When using this process to reach out to someone else, this is called attunement. Resonance comes with both the awareness of bodily sensations and attunement to the other. It is a process where we sense our embodied reactions towards the other and how what the other person brings also resonates inside us as this is an intimate process, and it may bring unexpectedly strong feelings when discussing sexuality.

When entering the erotic field (Clemmens, 2012), we often experience a powerful type of energy. The difficulties experienced in entering this energy field are often related to our cultural taboos, our fears of being accused of misconduct, the attitudes held towards sexuality in our family or religion, gender differences and sexual orientation, and our own sexual experiences and traumas. On the other hand, only through allowing ourselves to enter this zone may we be able to understand the nature of emerging sexuality in an embodied relational situation and thus support clients in gaining more awareness, as is indeed the main goal of gestalt therapy (Yontef, 1993).

Most of the time, entering this field has nothing to do with abuse and, as my earlier personal examples show, can bring insights into the therapeutic work. The ground for this work is, however, deeply embedded in societal dynamics that include heteronormativity or homonormativity (reactions to heteronormativity that ignore or criticise heterosexual identity).

4.1.3 Homophobia without homophobes

The title of this section is a paraphrase of the book entitled *Racism without Racists* by Bonilla-Silva (2006), which suggests that contemporary racism is often hidden and that most of us would not agree with being labelled a racist, and yet we exhibit occasional racist behaviours. In my work, I experience people who are both openly and subtly homophobic (see examples in the autoethnographic parts earlier and later in this chapter), but could it be that each of us embodies a degree of homophobia (or heterophobia)?

> Despite queer's interest in a politics of identity that seeks to consider bodies as mobile and fluid, these movements can never escape the territorializations of identity norms because they are always in relation to heteronormative coding and the overall arboreal organization of bodies that are directed inwards.
>
> (Ruffolo, 2012, p. 53)

As it is impossible to avoid homophobia in the heteronormative world in which we live, it is important that therapists have the space and conditions to be able to discuss and discover this. Some counselling and psychotherapy training enable this.

We live in a heteronormative world designed to support traditionally understood families, relationships, and romances. In fact, out of our awareness we may even exclude others in order to feel safer within our own sexual and gender identity. Salih writes that "a heterosexual matrix [. . .] has a vested interest in preserving its own stability and coherence at the expense of 'other' identities" (2002, p. 76). She suggests that "othering" is a process that enables us to feel more comfortable with who we are or think we should appear to be, and this chapter shows an example of how this is embodied. Embodied heteronormativity is a process which restricts or modifies the erotic field due to processes that escape awareness in relationships with people not representing our usually sexually preferred gender. Heteronormativity is not a phenomenon that belongs to an individual, but a social process that we all have been both victims and perpetrators of. It is, in fact, a collective gestalt that holds a dynamic polarity. Many members of the LGBTQI communities are embedded in this process often due to internalised oppression (a process in which the oppressed exhibit behaviours of the oppressors). The heteronormative processes are even more powerful processes in establishments and have permeated psychology and psychotherapy for decades.

4.1.4 Heteronormativity in psychotherapy between acceptance and abuse

Heteronormativity in psychotherapy has taken different forms. Initially, homosexuality was classified as a mental disorder (Committee on Nomenclature and Statistics of the American Psychiatric Association, 1968), and mainstream psychoanalytic training did not accept openly gay trainees. In the last 20 years, heteronormativity in psychotherapy took two polarities: from homohysteric (Anderson, 2009) attacks on homosexuality, such as in conversion pseudotherapies, and in the critique of gender studies to the collective silence found in most therapeutic establishments. I believe this silence is caused by lingering homophobia, but also uncertainties related to touch, sexuality, and gender identification.

In 1952, homosexuality became a mental disorder according to the second edition of the Diagnostic and Statistical Manual (Clarke, Ellis and Riggs, 2010, p. 12; Committee on Nomenclature and Statistics of the American Psychiatric Association, 1968) and it was criminalised in the UK until 1967 (Zachary, 2001, p. 490). From the beginning of psychoanalysis, homosexuality was treated as a psychological disturbance. Most psychoanalysts treated it either as a sexual deviation (Twomey, 2003, pp. 9–10), *fear of castration*, *penis envy*, or as a defence against psychosis, neurosis, or both (Holland, 1992, pp. 89–92). Openly gay people were not even accepted onto psychoanalytic training until the 1980s (Twomey, 2003, p. 9). Although, these attitudes have changed (see later in this chapter), some of the prejudices remain.

About ten years ago, in one of the most cited homophobic texts in Poland written by the head of a Polish psychotherapy institute, Milska-Wrzosińska (2002) argued that gay people should not expect society to support them and reinforced many stereotypes of lesbian, gay, and transgender people. Amongst the stereotypes, Milska-Wrzosińska blames overprotective or inaccessible mothers in the development of the gay male identity. She refers to her successful cases of helping such men to come back on track to heterosexuality. However, apart from this, she does not take a stance towards conversion pseudotherapy (therapy aiming at converting clients' sexual orientation to heterosexual). In a commentary on this article and in response to a wave of critique, she claimed that she had the courage to say what most therapists actually think (Tomasik, 2004, p. 74). Although this might be believed to be an isolated example of homophobia, some research evidences that the majority of psychotherapists in the UK have not received any training around gender and sexuality discourse at all (Davies and Aykroyd, 2002), and it is likely that a similar dynamic occurs in other countries. Typically, under heteronormative assumptions, homosexuality is pathologised and assessed regarding its aetiology, while heterosexual identity is left unanalysed. There is another prejudice embedded in this thinking. In a survey undertaken in 2001 in the UK of 218 members of the British Confederation of Psychotherapists, 64% responded that their clients' homosexuality was central to the difficulties they presented (Bartlett, King and Phillips, 2001). Although obvious that heteronormativity had a severe impact on mental wellbeing, the responders seemed to suggest that it was homosexuality itself that was the problem.

Similar assumptions support gay conversion pseudotherapies, which aim to bring homosexuals "back to" heterosexuality, believed to be the only "natural" and "healthy" state. Recent research on conversion pseudotherapy (Dickinson et al., 2014) evidenced that this treatment was ineffective and abusive. In the last few years, the UK psychotherapy associations, the British Association for Counselling and Psychotherapy and the United Kingdom Council for Psychotherapy, condemned conversion pseudotherapies and informed their members that conducting conversion pseudotherapy is in breach of the psychotherapeutic code of ethics (Memorandum of Understanding on Conversion Therapy in the UK, 2015). In 2018 the European Parliament condemned but did not delegalise conversion pseudotherapy (Duffy, 2018). A US-based organisation, Exodus International, closed down and issued an apology for all the abuse they participated in (Zand, 2015). With some organisations still engaging in this activity, for example The National Association for the Research and Therapy of Homosexuality, it remains a stronghold of legal homophobia and homohysteria in psychology (Wikipedia, 2017). Most psychotherapeutic establishments today support clients in accepting rather than changing their sexual identity (Memorandum of Understanding on Conversion Therapy in the UK, 2015). Nevertheless, remnants of homophobia certainly remain in the mainstream of counselling and psychotherapy.

I refer to the situation in Poland not only because I follow their heteronormative discourse, but also because it is an example of a country where homophobia is supported by a large part of society and the government. The Polish example shows collective gestalts that have been dormant in many countries and can be reactivated. Recently in Poland, it is not just LGBTQI communities which are being attacked, but also gender researchers and writers. These homohysteric attacks appear at the same time as researchers identify homosexuality as the main reason for social exclusion in Poland (Hearn and Pringle, 2006, p. 138). In 2017, the Polish right-wing Prime Minister Beata Szydło gave the highest order of service to the country to an organisation that is dedicated to conversion pseudotherapy (Ambroziak, 2017). My Polish gestalt colleagues, including Daniel Bąk, Kamila Biały, and Piotr Mierkowski, have been involved in direct actions to save Polish clients and psychotherapists from this demagogy.

One of the most common techniques in conversion pseudotherapy is touch therapy. In this technique "patients" are invited to cuddle the therapist in the same way that I did during the therapy described earlier.

In this video, Cohen (CNN, 2006), a person who claims he used to be gay, offers a man's touch, which he believes is what all gay man want instead of sexual contact. The level of denial of how this situation may be constructed sexually contrasts with my sense of the importance to express and feel acceptance of my same-sex desire for my therapist Tom. I feel very lucky that I was able to explore my feelings and sensations with an embodied non-homophobic therapist. A therapist less comfortable with men's touch or sexual intimacy in general could bring about shame in a client in a similar situation.

In more severe cases, therapists can be openly homophobic or homohysterical (Anderson, 2009). As reported by some of my clients who went through conversion pseudotherapies, the most difficult part of it is that the pseudotherapist himself often represses his same-sex sexual desires, hence what they call touch therapy is often a form of sexual exchange. Pseudotherapists touch clients with denial that this relationship may also have mutual erotic feelings. It is a border-making process where embodied sensations are not given the right name. "Pathologically serious are those traumatic confusions that are [. . .] placed at the level of corporeal sensations (Id-function of the Self)", writes Salonia (2016, p. 25). Having explored the spectrum of homophobia in psychotherapy, let's look at how it occurs within therapeutic modalities.

4.1.5 Heteronormativity in contemporary psychoanalysis and gestalt therapy

In the last 20 years, psychoanalytic theory underwent a massive change. Freud's incest taboo, exemplified by the Oedipus complex, was criticised by Butler (2011) and Benjamin (1996). Butler (2011) suggested that the taboo of homosexuality can be even greater, remaining a difficult subject to discuss even within psychoanalysis. Contemporary psychoanalytic therapists talk about "triangular relationships" (e.g. a child with her two fathers). They argue that relationships happen in triangles and this will be regardless of parental gender and sexual orientation (Benjamin, 1996). They believe that with incest taboo, some sense of crime takes place within a triangular parent and child relationship: "to go back to the first triangle, for homosexuals there will be some sin, some crime and some illness, just as is the case for heterosexuals" (Zachary, 2001, p. 492). Heterosexual and homosexual taboos are not the same; this sense of *crime, illness*, and *sin* has a different flavour that impacts how they occur later in a therapeutic relationship. Yet, they are both infused by the difficulty in discussing mutuality or the erotic field.

When the relational theory started to impact psychoanalysis, sessions quickly became desexualised (Renn, 2013). Although, before, psychoanalysts were treating the sexual drive as one of the two main motivating factors for their patients seeking therapy, after introducing an authentic relational presence into the room, sexuality soon became a taboo that also appears to be often reduced to transference (Renn, 2013). There are also exceptions to this taboo (Slavin et al., 2004). Similar silencing occurs in gestalt psychotherapy training.

Although in contrast with much early psychoanalysis and other therapeutic modalities, gestalt therapy accepted LGBTQI communities into psychotherapy training from its foundation; a discussion on gender and sexual orientation, however, does not play a part in the regular curriculum. The fact that gestalt therapists do not often discuss homophobia is probably a sign that it exists. Not only is homophobia an embodied field phenomenon, but this phenomenon has a unique role to play in each relationship. Although there is some literature available on gender (Amendt-Lyon, 2008; Flansted-Jensen, 2008; Novack, Park and Friedman, 2013), working with transgender clients (Bennett, 2010; Fallon, 2012; Kolmannskog, 2014; Hawley, 2011), and sexual orientation in gestalt psychotherapy (see literature review in Amendt-Lyon, 2013), the discussion on embodied heteronormativity is limited. Flansted-Jensen (2008) introduces the concept of gender as something that we do rather than something we are (Butler, 2011) as compatible with the gestalt approach, and encourages playful experimentation as a way to dismantle fixed genders in the companies she works with. Johnson (2014) and O'Shea (2000) explain the necessity of attending to the themes of sexual diversity in training and therapy to change attitudes of both students and trainers. Kepner notices: "my own view of [gender and sexuality in] Gestalt theory is that it is much ado about too little. Our theory articulates too little in relation to specific content areas such as gender and sexuality" (2008, p. 126). A limited discussion implies the difficulty of addressing embodied heteronormativity. As the autobiographical part evidences, issues around sexual orientation are not only something clients bring to the room but also therapists. Again, as with psychoanalysis, I think the resistance I experienced to exploring my felt erotic sense with some of my clients was not only related to an embodied homophobia, but also to the embodied societal dynamics of *sin, crime*, and *illness*, which affect current psychotherapy.

4.2　Homophobia in the practice of the embodied gestalt therapist

4.2.1　Embodied heteronormativity – phenomenology and bodywork

There are ways of attending to felt phenomenological sensations, such as mindfulness or focusing (Gendlin, 2010); however, staying true to a gestalt methodology, I have applied two phenomenological analyses of experiences. The first one, which I call *embodying*, is close to the classical psychological phenomenology of attending to sensuous experiences through suspension of beliefs (*epoché*), describing them, and treating them with equal importance (horizontalisation) (Spinelli, 2005). The second step I call *resonating*, which focuses on the interactions with others and with culture, for example, the noticing of embodied resonance. Before I describe my own experiences, I would like to invite the reader to experience an embodied experiment that I often suggest during my workshops and conference presentations on this subject. I offer a version of this experiment to the trainee and to the experienced psychotherapists only once I feel there is a level of intimacy established within the group. I disclose that it is an experiment, aimed at exploring participants' sexualities and they should opt out at any moment that they may feel uneasy or even confused. Furthermore, I suggest that some people may already find it difficult when a male presenter invites them to an exploration of sexuality, and I leave some space for this to be discussed. I do not recommend this exercise to people who have experienced any post-traumatic stress related to a sexual incident. I outline the following experiment and invite you to follow it in your mind.

> Imagine meeting face to face with a stranger. For a moment, close your eyes and imagine feeling the presence of this person next to you. Let yourself tune in to any erotic sensations; be aware of them and their energetic wishes and desires. Now look at this person in your mind and pick an element of that person which might attract you in this embodied erotic way. If there are many elements, just pick one – for example, an eyebrow, a piece of cloth, or the way the person sits. For a moment, let yourself be mesmerised and attracted by this element. Notice what quality of sensations you experience; notice both the feelings towards attraction, eroticism, curiosity, as well as those feelings which take you away from, for example, feelings of strangeness, inappropriateness, or danger. Notice both and try not to judge them at

this stage, but simply keep noticing. Now, if it helps, take a moment and note down your observations.

Suggesting this experiment towards the end of seminars I have led at conferences, when I feel we have already established a safe, non-judgemental space, has brought some interesting insights. The direct exploration of sexuality between men, women, and trans people from a spectrum of sexual orientation allowed explorations of intimacy and attraction. For example, two heterosexual men spoke about the need to be cuddled and close physically with one another; two heterosexual women allowed themselves to explore female attraction, noticing how different it was to what they have usually experienced with men. It was non-predatory, one commented. At the same time, participants reported that they do not usually allow themselves to explore this level of intimacy with either their clients or friends. Furthermore, this exploration allowed other societal taboos about sexuality to surface, in particular those of ageing and disability. Some senior disabled psychotherapists reported not allowing themselves to feel like objects of sexual desire or attraction, assuming a client's sexual needs or fantasies would not be directed towards them. We all have ways of embodying shame that may prevent us from noticing the important erotic vitality that will at some point appear in our therapy rooms.

Of course psychotherapy is not a space for fulfilment of erotic needs, but the safe expression of them is an opportunity for greater intimacy and powerful psychotherapeutic work that includes sexuality, gender, abuse, joy, fulfilment, excitement, and other areas that we and our clients may associate with erotic vitality.

These explorations in the workshop inspired me to ask myself similar questions and notice how I embody heteronormativity. Outcomes of these explorations are presented next.

4.2.1.1 Embodying

When I sense homophobia in myself, I notice a great deal of awareness of my upper body. I breathe deeply into my lungs and often experience clarity of my mind. I feel capable of doing a lot and I have waves of energy where I feel like doing something manual with my hands. I have quick thinking and responses; I feel some pleasure in that as I interpret it as being strong. My pelvis is locked backwards, and I feel tightness in my lower abdomen. I do not feel much in my genitals; however, I sense I am standing firmly on my legs.

When letting myself be sexual and intimate, I notice how I immediately slow down. I also experience some shame. I am much more anxious as my yearning for intimacy makes me more aware of people around me. I breathe into my stomach and then lungs. I sense my genitals and notice how I sit heavily on my pelvis. My thoughts are a bit more confused and slower. I sense my face and feel vulnerable, knowing that it is showing more of my feelings now, and I am much more visible. I feel more human.

My heteronormativity is creating a distance from both my feelings and my body in general, which includes the erotic. It is a feature of a strong heterosexual presence so that it rests on desensitisation (Thomas, 2008). It requires an embodiment of certainty. Brothers (2007) believes that acts of certainty are often related to trauma. The state of being certain shows only how little space is left in the field for discussion, ambiguity and diverse perspectives. While my heteronormativity leads to certainty, the Socratic "I know that I know nothing" is a state that psychotherapists should maintain or even cultivate (Staemmler, 1997) with their clients. My second example from the large groups shows my shifting position on immigration from certain to inclusive through the work on my personal trauma (see Section 2.2.2). However, slowing down and letting ourselves feel the lack of certainty brings difficult feelings, especially when it comes to gender identity.

The shame I experience when slowing down may be related to the fact that shame is a natural feeling associated with becoming intimate (Jacobs, 1996), but may also relate to this sense of *crime, sin,* and *illness* (Zachary, 2001) and of simply becoming aware of one's sexuality. If sexuality is related to intimacy and deepening interpersonal connection as much as withdrawal of sexuality reduces intimacy, heteronormativity impacts the way we resonate kinaesthetically (Frank and Barre, 2011) in relationships.

4.2.1.2 Resonating

Alexander Lowen (1994) described "rigid character structure" as a fixed embodiment of a sexually charged and confusing childhood. Rigid character structure was an effect of a field where there was no permission to experience sexuality or there was some tension around the experience of sexuality. Natural attempts of a child to be close to a parent with all aspects of his or her personality were rejected. If a rigid character structure is an effect of the field of the family in this case, what effect on the body does a social field of heteronormativity have? My reminiscence of my pelvis locked back; my way of focusing my eyes on women in my childhood, and even now; and my deflated sense of resignation (the cool boys at that time were inflated) have all impacted on the way I have engaged and contributed to the creation of an enduring relational theme (Jacobs, 2011, 2017). Heteronormativity is a strong social process (even stronger when unspoken) which creates a field that influences our embodiment and our sensual processes.

A psychoanalyst and feminist, Susie Orbach (2010), suggests exploring our embodiment from the point of view of the body. What she means is to start the analysis from the question of, "why our body needs to be the way it is" rather than from, "what it is about the mind that we want to embody". In this light, I am drawn to examine my own gender ambiguity during my childhood and the fact that people sometimes mistook me for a girl.

Although initially I enjoyed playing with different expressions of genders (see Figure 4.3 earlier), later I felt ashamed and confused when acting girlishly. I am aware that this confusion served as a substitute for something else. The biggest confusion for me in my childhood, overall, was uncertainty about the survival of my family as a unit. Often, arguments at my home would create much anxiety for me. At this time, however, I was more worried about my body, gender identity, and sexuality. I recreated a familiar situation and feeling to move away from my deepest fear that my family will collapse. Also, I had the insecurity that I felt that my parents would have preferred a girl. Initially, they did not even have a boy's name for me when I was born; a girl's name had been chosen. Whilst at this stage I am not able to identify my mother's real reasons behind her preference, I think I have more clarity about my father's. He always seemed to be fearful of each occurrence of men's aggression. I think this related to his experience of the Second World War and even before that, growing up during the growth of the National Socialist German Workers' Party (NSDAP) in Germany. I imagine, for my father, my emerging maleness was difficult.

4.2.2 Heteronormative contacting

Gestalt therapists are therapists who are concerned with contact, while paying attention to what style of contact we use in a certain moment. In this chapter, I describe various styles of contact (Joyce and Sills, 2009), such as deflection, projection, introjection, confluence, and desensitisation, which might be experienced when working with homophobia. I also make observations related to phenomenology and to field theory.

Deflection in gestalt is understood as an avoidance manoeuvre, a sudden change of a topic or of experience of feelings. Practically, it can manifest as unexpected laughter, sudden questioning, or just a change of topic to be discussed. When applying this to heteronormativity, I have noticed that it often occurs in my therapeutic relationships with men, when intimacy is about to happen and that Eastern European men have been blunter in acting it out than Western men.

4.2.2.1 2013

A Romanian client, Anton, was a man whose father died when he was five. Since that time, he followed the "real man's" path without questioning it. He played in a semi-professional football team, completed a degree in construction, and was managing a successful large-scale construction site where women appeared only in the canteen. He was aware of his father's deficits, and when we came closer to talking about his feelings of abandonment by his father, I looked into his eyes and was surprised to see not tears, but sparks. He smiled. "This is so much like faggots", he said. "Or sensitive men", I jumped in, perhaps slightly too quickly, offering him a male alternative and also ignoring his homophobia.

As I worked with him, I began to realise that he did not have suitable ways of expressing his feelings when it came to coming into contact with his grief. He was moving towards his grief, and then homophobia was the only way he knew how to manage it. Homophobia is sometimes used to prevent intimacy between men. A strong straight male identity is often linked to disembodiment (Thomas, 2008). McCormack (2012, p. 72) notices how homophobia reduces tactility between boys, and I also believe that the impacts are much greater for both the development of an aware sexuality and for intimacy between men. This was confirmed in a number of workshops that I facilitated for psychotherapists, where heterosexual male participants found themselves more tactile with other heterosexual men when bisexuality was allowed. Anderson (2009) calls it "homosociality", a term that describes an openness towards bisexuality and invites new expressions of masculinities.

More tender and loving feelings quite often challenge me more than more overtly sexual topics, and this is something that other men have also reported (Gabbard, 1996, p. 140). Although it was similar to my experience with my male therapist, where my homophobia was keeping me from the ability to experience intimacy, when I was working with my first gay client, I did not feel ready to experience my sexual feelings with him.

> We know that many people have same-sex experiences or erotic feelings during their adult life. It could also be that earlier same-sex sexual experience or crushes perhaps in adolescence or early adulthood have left the therapist with unresolved issues. The different choices they made may impede their availability to work at relational depth with the lesbian, gay or bisexual client for fear of being seduced off the "straight and narrow" path.
>
> (Davies and Aykroyd, 2002, p. 230)

My experience of facilitating the workshops described earlier taught me that we all are capable of experiencing sexual feeling or embodied sexual countertransference even with a group of people we would not normally orient ourselves towards. "The psyche is an entity that is irreducibly bisexual, representational, and symbolic," writes Fogel (2009, p. 231). This hypothesis invites therapists to pay attention and they may be surprised as to why, with certain clients or groups of clients, they may seem less able to connect through their own sexual body resonance even though their clients may experience sexual feelings. Although sexuality constitutes an important part of life, the awareness of erotic feelings is not always present in the consulting room. It can be noted that this awareness may also be affected by homonormative experiences for gay therapists. At the same time, heteronormativity (or homonormativity) is not the only reason for a lack of sexual body resonance in therapy; working with severely depressed clients, for instance, such feelings might often not be available at the initial stages of therapy.

Heteronormativity spoken and unspoken may be a way of deflecting from intimacy and sexuality in the counselling room by both the client and the therapist. It could be a deflection that is hard to notice and work with, and could remain mostly unspoken. Field-oriented gestalt therapists are invited to unpack cultural assumptions both theoretically and practically. By exploring gender roles within their own social identification, therapists create a safe space for exploring erotic feelings in their consulting rooms.

One of the oldest concepts about heteronormativity is that it is a projection (attributing to someone else elements of our own thoughts, feelings, and behaviours). For example, a woman who is homophobic may condemn gay people, due to her being uneasy about her own sexuality or sexual orientation. I think this is particularly applicable to people brought up in a society dominated by a culture and religion that does not allow the exploration of sexuality freely (Ranke-Heinemann, 1994). In Poland all attempts to explore my sexuality were classified as a sin, and the only sexual language I knew before my 20s was a mixture of vulgar, sexually explicit street language and guilt-dominated Catholic confession-like statements.

Analysing my own childhood, I experienced much fear of being projected onto and being scapegoated, and so I tried to attract women to get out of this situation. When working with Anton, my quick reaction, trying to create the option of "emotional men", was not only an attempt to give him an option but another way of me rescuing myself from being labelled as a "faggot" once again. There is an invitation to confluence there. Confluence is a state when two or more people become one and see themselves as more alike than different. The heteronormative confluence that men are all alike contributed to how I had felt excluded during my childhood. The exclusion was delivered through identification with the terms, or slurs, of me being "gay" or "a girl". Unexplored collective gestalts offer a sense of false belonging (confluence) with groups that share the same prejudice along with the sense of detachment and emptiness as shown in my autoethnographic examples.

The attitude which links gender with sexuality is also part of the heteronormative assumptions which, as Hawley (2011) evidenced, are still leaking into psychotherapeutic practice. This clearly links with the introjections (unexamined beliefs) about what a "real man" (or "real woman") should be. Most magazines, television shows, and films reinforce societal beliefs about how men and women should be. Only recently, some films for children have started to cast women not only as princesses or mothers, but also as warriors and politicians. If it comes to men, the homohysteria leads significantly to a reduction in touch and the possibility to be tactile (Anderson, 2009).

4.3 Heteronormativity and touch

The introjection of stereotypical beliefs in therapy and society lead to concepts of shame in gestalt therapy, understood as a lack of support from within the environment that is both internal and external. Shame is closely related to belonging as, according to relational gestalt therapy, we are all wired for connection and belonging (Jacobs, 2009). When our sense of belonging is endangered we choose an available option to defend against it; for example, for me with the group of boys in my childhood, the choice was either to sink into shame or to defend with homophobia. Showing I was straight was an unsuccessful attempt to belong that was only worked through in my therapy with Tom (see Section 4.1.1.3), but even then, it came with a great deal of shame.

Tom allowed me also to challenge my prejudice with regards to touch in my therapy with him. Others might not. For various reasons, touch is not encouraged in gestalt therapy in England. Despite the fact that a reduction of physical distance in a therapeutic space can create some cause for concern, as Eiden (2011) puts it for example, "avoidance of hostility through collusive gratification, and re-enactment of abuse through invasive techniques" (p. 49), touch also has much to offer in psychotherapy.

> Touch will usually evoke a bodily response from the other; it is an essential form of communication and we speak and listen through our hands. Mere hand to hand contact can reveal distinct and unique patterns of personal psyche-soma dynamics. Touch may be warm, mechanical or withdrawn, evoke sensations, feelings and inter-personal dynamics, or elicit involuntary or disavowed motor intentions.
>
> (Warnecke, 2011, p. 236)

Although body psychotherapists say that touch can help clients to reduce pain, facilitate biochemical change, and help them to feel soothed and nurtured (Eiden, 1998, p. 5), in line with the paradoxical theory of change (Beisser, 1970), gestalt therapists do not explicitly want to change a client's state. Touch in gestalt therapy is a way to connect and to attend to how we connect. Through touch, clients can increase their awareness of their needs, feelings, and relationships which, according to the paradoxical theory of change, leads to more acceptance of who we are and, in turn, often to change. With so many advantages of touch in psychotherapy, I was frustrated that we were not taught how to use touch during my training in England, and the experience of touch which helped me to work through my homophobia (see Section 4.1.1.1) took place only when I left my gestalt therapist to work with a body orientated psychotherapist. I believe there are several reasons why touch is not popular in gestalt therapy in England:

- Cultural differences – during my training in Poland trainee therapists would practise how to attend through touch to clients; during my training in England, touch was not discussed explicitly and if it was, it was mostly discouraged.
- Fear of litigation – with no witness in one-to-one therapy, psychotherapists fear they might be accused of sexual abuse.
- Abuse – lack of professional boundaries during the beginnings of gestalt therapy led to some clients feeling violated by their therapists between the 1950s and 1980s. However, even now touch may be detrimental to some of our clients, and therapists require special training to understand their own potential to be harmful (see Chapter 5).
- Traumatisation – related to the previous point, touch is a strong and intimate intervention, and so has a potential to deepen the trauma for some clients and needs to be used and offered with much awareness.
- Fear of sex, homophobia, and heterophobia – societal phobias have a strong effect on psychotherapy, which likes to believe it is counter-cultural, and hence not influenced by societal norms.

All these leads to a culture of retroflection in the UK, with therapists holding back through their non-responsiveness, and through their interpretations and embodied responses they may often shame clients who feel the need for touch (for example, a handshake, hug, or holding a hand). Although it may seem that I want to encourage gestalt practitioners to use touch, we are not yet ready to do so. Lack of training, cultural awareness of touch, and discussions on societal phobias in our training thus far does not create practitioners who are equipped in non-judgemental and open ways to attend to touch within therapy. What is required is cultural change in our training and in our community towards touch, and the gradual building of support through workshops, in supervision, and via publications. Although gestalt therapy does not have a formalised definition of health (Bar-Yoseph Levine, 2012, p. 3), freedom to experiment was always at the heart of it. In the following section, I describe the similarity between new materialism and gestalt definitions of health.

4.4 Body discourse and desire

Despite coming from different philosophical traditions, gestalt therapy theory seems to have a close relationship to new materialism, which was a theoretical base for some of the theories presented in this book (see Section 6.2). Both theories see embodied process (gender and sexuality included) as an outcome of a sort of negotiation between various involved matters (an individual, culture, society, physicality).

> Gayness (or straightness) is neither produced from causes – whether physiological, genetic, neurological, or sociological – nor is it the consequence of a free choice among equally appealing given alternatives. It is the enactment of a freedom that can refuse to constrain sexuality and sexual partners to any given function, purpose, or activity and that makes sexuality an open invention even as it carries the burden of biological, cultural, and individual construction.
>
> (Grosz, 2010, p. 153)

The *enactment of freedom* with a *burden* is exactly what is needed to enable more gender and sexual fluidity in the psychotherapeutic process, and the embodied lively erotic energy is the drive that can phenomenologically guide us towards this direction. Deleuze and Guattari ask: "Why such a dreary parade of sucked-dry, catatonicized, vitrified, sewn-up bodies, when the [body] is also full of gaiety, ecstasy, and dance?" (1987, p. 150). Deleuze and Guattari (1987) show the contrast between keeping the vivid and ecstatic energy at bay, creating both safe and depleted embodiments, and ecstatic, dancing bodies that are free to explore. Gestalt therapists apply aesthetic criteria in diagnosis, including clarity, liveliness, harmony, grace, and fluidity (Robine, 2007, p. 12) to define healthy functioning as a form of phenomenological diagnosis. The freedom to experiment and feel the liveliness of the body is an erotic experience, claims O'Shea (2016). There is a clear link between the erotic energy in the therapeutic room and the freedom to experiment in a performative way (Butler, 2011) with the new ways of being.

What Butler (2011) means by performative can be defined in terms of gestalt experimentation. Each act of enacting, imagining, sitting in a new chair, trying a behaviour, or rehearing an old introject is a performative act. The body of the therapist needs to be free to embody various sexualities, and it also needs to be trained in the possible prejudices and abuses we may carry.

Although sexual abuse of clients takes place in psychotherapy (Samuels, 2016), the repression of eroticism is a major contributor to the lack of awareness and maturity of relationally co-emergent sexuality. "The erotic is often messy. A mature therapeutic relationship must also have the capacity to be messy", argues Cornell (2003, p. 100). Developing the idea of sexuality being repressed by modern institutions (Foucault, 1990), Deleuze and Guattari notice how psychoanalysts had taken the role of *priests* and how through their theories desire is pathologised, and hence undermined (1987, p. 154). Samuels (2003) notices that the taboo about therapists not having sex with clients comes from an impulse that therapists have. The art of working with sexuality in therapy lies in freeing the liveliness of this desire in a way that is not abusive physically or mentally to our clients. This book is an attempt to free psychotherapeutic desire both from the fear of addressing sexuality as well as heteronormative assumptions present in psychotherapeutic practice. Ruffolo argues that queer theorists should not engage in polarised discussions, but question the underlying politics:

> In other words, the queer/heteronormative dyad halts queer politics when the politics of queer is predominantly concerned with disrupting heteronormative structures. Post-queer rhizomatic politics is about deterritorializing politics itself rather than opposing an a priori structure. This project is one line of flight amongst many that can remap contemporary politics as we know it today.
>
> (2012, p. 54)

By questioning the assumption behind some psychotherapeutic politics and deconstructing introjects around sexuality in the therapy room, I would like to disrupt structures that restrict sexuality in psychotherapy. It is the embodied phenomenology of desire and eroticism that can lead us to dismantle restrictive politics, as it did in my journey of reducing embodied heteronormativity. Paying attention to phenomenological sensations of desire in the consulting room and asking questions when this desire is not present or available should be a part of therapeutic work and is, in fact, a political statement in itself.

4.5 Conclusion

As for autoethnography, this chapter demonstrates how a single person's story just by itself creates a challenge to more traditional ways of understanding attraction and same-sex attraction in counselling and psychotherapy. The reversed chronological narration of my own story from low prejudices nowadays to high prejudices in the past tracks back my exploration of a here-and-now embodied phenomenon that occurred in my therapeutic practice with Marek. It is an invitation to consider how to present biographical writing to maximise its impact on the readers and explain theory through personal, and hopefully moving, examples. It is also a self-compassionate reflection on how to describe the conditions that created our prejudices.

I think it is important to create conditions in our lives in which we will be challenged to discover our prejudices, including heteronormativity. As in gestalt psychology, our needs shape the environment, our sexual needs and desires can make us blind towards some of the feelings and embodied sensations expressed in our consulting rooms. We need to find ways of talking about sexual needs and desires in a way that takes into consideration gender power dynamics and other possibilities of exploitation. As many gestalt therapists report not having any modules on sexual diversity in their training, it is evident how homophobia is present and unspoken. Discovering one's prejudices is an emotionally challenging process that requires certain conditions to occur (Gadamer, 2012).

Collective gestalts cannot be learned, at least not in a traditional way. What we can learn is how to increase our confidence when our identity is shaken; we can learn how to survive these moments of fear or shame and draw conclusions; how to be open for dialogue with relatively low defence and only a mild sense of safety. Collective gestalts are not states or achievements, but processes, ways of dialoguing both outside and inside (and between parts of ourselves). Furthermore, it is through the bravery of launching into unknown territory, exploring difference and allowing ourselves to show our ignorance, that we can grow. This chapter explored the beginning of my ongoing journey of ignorance related to my sexual identity. The journey between a higher and lower heteronormativity showed how my own homophobia was co-created and deconstructed through interpersonal and social factors. My sexual orientation moved from settled heterosexual toward what Braidotti (2011, p. 76) calls *nomadic*, i.e. not fixed, dualistic, oppositional, and context-dependent.

This chapter aims to challenge more traditional views about embodied sexual transference across sexual orientations. Since heteronormativity has been widespread in psychotherapeutic and psychoanalytic circles for many years, I hope to open a discussion about how it may still occur in our embodiment through personal attitudes and prejudices. Furthermore, I question and challenge the power of heteronormativity and psychotherapeutic fear of sexuality to inhibit desire. A "politics of becoming calls for a return to [the] productive flows of desire" (Ruffolo, 2012, p. 54). This chapter invites therapists to increase "the ability to play (in the Winnicottian sense) with varied gendered expressions of self without threat to sense of self" (Elise, 1998, p. 357). Although it is necessary to be open to the playful exploration of sexuality, it is only a gateway to deep relational attachment patterns embedded in any relationship. I believe more research on long-term attachment in same-sex therapeutic relationships is needed.

Similarly, the impact of culture on embodiment requires more attention. While in this chapter I have discussed the relationship between heteronormativity and desensitisation, the following chapter looks at how culture shapes gestalt training and produces enculturated bodies.

Chapter 5

(Un)related bodies

Collective gestalts that shape gestalt training

It is not possible to fully differentiate between the personal and the professional; one informs the other. The development of my practical skills and theoretical understandings are presented in this chapter in relation to my personal relationships and struggles on my way to becoming a gestalt therapist. Embedded in the culture of the trainings and the larger cultural milieu, collective gestalts moderate and are moderated by these struggles.

Ten years have passed between the two autoethnographic examples of the gestalt way of working presented later in this chapter. The experiences were recorded in two different countries: the first in Eastern Europe and the second in Western Europe and by two almost completely different men: myself during my university studies, and myself as a certified gestalt psychotherapist. The elements which separate those two men include many years of training as a psychotherapist and many hours of individual and group therapy, the loss of my father, some other life crises, an emigration to the UK, and many other impactful experiences that created the therapist I am becoming. Analysis of the two experiences, inspired by bioenergetics (a type of therapy that focuses on techniques releasing emotional tension through physical manipulation such as massage), gestalt therapy (a type of body therapy that I experienced in Poland), and Embodied Relational Gestalt therapy (which I studied in the UK and the USA) show an evolution of my thinking about group therapy facilitation. The story of my own becoming a gestalt therapist is shown in this chapter in reference to how gestalt therapy evolved in the last 50 years. The relational attitude in gestalt therapy (Hycner and Jacobs, 1995; Yontef, 2009) is presented as a motor, driving changes and providing the theoretical background for current developments in gestalt therapy. The final section presents a shift in gestalt group therapy approach.

The main differences between the two models are related to the position of the therapist and the concept of "co-creation", which believes that all themes in therapy are co-created or co-emergent. This shift could be compared to the onto-epistemological change between materialism grounded in the objectivistic division between matter, and the intellect and the new materialism that accentuates the discursive and situational nature of matter (Barad, 2007) (more in Chapter 6).

Embodied Relational Gestalt considers the therapist's body as a necessary and important part of therapy, and for gaining insights about the client and the therapist. Throughout this text, I will call this model "relational" or "dialogic", as it is concerned with how client and therapist are constantly interrelated. A clinical comparison between the two examples in this chapter is not possible because neither of the examples is a detailed case study. In an autoethnographic sense, it is a story of a journey, both personal and professional, rather than a comparison of the two groups I attended.

Describing the early gestalt body therapy model, I will be referring to my experiences from the beginning of the millennium, understanding that the pure model, as evidenced in the example, is not commonly used nowadays. However, it is my belief and experience that remnants of this style are still present both in teaching and in facilitating group therapy worldwide.

5.1 Autoethnography

Autoethnography and, more specifically, autophenomenography (see Section 7.1) aims to provide critical as well as rigorous descriptions of experiences generated through attention to phenomenological sensations (Allen-Collinson, 2011, 2013). In this chapter, I present two experiences, each describing a piece of body psychotherapy. The first (Section 5.1.2) was experienced by myself during my training in gestalt psychotherapy in Poland; the second (Section 5.1.3) is an example from my own work as a gestalt body therapist and trainer in the UK.

Various elements of Section 5.1.2 have been changed to preserve the anonymity of the therapist and the group attendees. As consent may have been difficult to obtain due to the critical attitude towards this method of working, I have decided not to request it. It is important that gestalt therapists reflect critically on some of the methods applied, and describing a training workshop from 15 years ago that has been anonymised does not raise serious ethical concerns (see Section 7.4).

5.1.1 Field theory is transference

Bioenergetic and gestalt-inspired body therapy (bioenergetic gestalt) recognises elements of field theory (Lewin, 1952) as it states that reactions to other members of the group are from different field conditions and hence should be worked on. Furthermore, they notice that an individual piece of work affects other participants, often creating themes in/for a group. What is being ignored in this approach is the co-creation of all themes together by both the clients as well as the therapist. In the embodied relational model, fields of the therapist and clients meet, and they impact each other. Experiences from fields outside of the therapy room are recreated and reactivated in a group or a therapeutic relationship, and can be changed through awareness paid to the here-and-now interpersonal relationships.

In the first group, I described when a female member stated that, following my cathartic work, she felt frightened. The therapist immediately interpreted it as a transference, or an experience from different field conditions, and offered to work on it with the woman in the middle. Her fear of me shouting and pushing other men and the mattress (see Figure 5.1) is seen as a distortion of reality rather than an attunement to reality, and there is an interesting argument behind it, that of transference. There is a positivistic assumption behind the classical transference theory, while field theory is based on an intersubjective epistemology (co-construction, or better, co-emergency). If the therapist treated the complaint of this group participant as an insight into the field of the group that she had co-created, she would then have to give consideration to how we had created an environment in which some people felt afraid. We as a group would have had to answer questions about our need to scare people, or feel strong or even superior. In line with field theory, relational therapy gives attention not only to individuals but also to the reactions other people have to them, and how we participate and co-create relationships and the overall atmosphere of a group.

To truly embrace what field theory can offer, therapists must be able to engage both their hearts and minds, and to study power relationships within the room as well as critically examine their own political, cultural, sexual, and theoretical positions. Wheeler (2006) states that it is the field itself that is a source of healing. This can only happen when group dynamics are explored along with hearing people's experiences from the past.

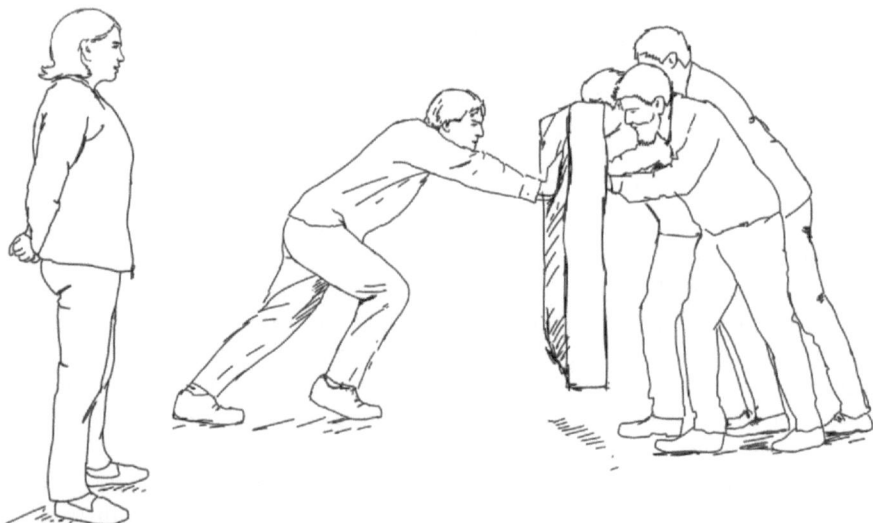

Figure 5.1 Bioenergetics and gestalt-inspired body therapy in practice: pushing the mattress
Source: Anna Taterka (2017a).

5.1.2 Example 1: bioenergetics and gestalt-inspired body therapy

I was 23 years old and studied philosophy in a city devastated by an extensive mining industry. Drilling took place beneath the city itself. Communist investment in mining was faster than the city could cope with and hence, not only was the air polluted, but also some of the streets had collapsed. I was hanging out with a group of creative students and my lifestyle was one of drinking, partying, and occasional drunken dances at a local jazz club, all carefully masking my depression and anxieties related to attending university. I was often too tired to get up in the morning, so I skipped most of my classes and went to the university students' union at around 3 p.m. My girlfriend at that time, Mariola, was a kind and tender person far away from my world and …I did not treat her very well. I was busy with my "cool" friends and I made her feel unwanted. I decided to study gestalt therapy as I needed to have a profession beyond philosophy, and I found it to be more interesting than anything else I had studied. A significant part of the gestalt training was via group therapy, and in the middle of the first year we attended an intensive five days (9 a.m. to 7 p.m.) of group therapy. A few years before this experience, I had been in individual therapy in the same centre for about two years.

The residential group therapy was a mixture of individual work in the middle ("hot seat") and group exercises. We started with exercises and focused on our own bodies, through breathing, moving around, and shouting. When exhausted from shouting, I began coughing up phlegm and the therapist explained to me that these were my introjects (unexamined assumptions which I "swallowed" from other people) and now I needed to spit them out. So, we spat into tissues as we lay on the floor and shouted, engaging, using our diaphragms. After a while, I noticed that my voice had deepened and that I was experiencing pain in my throat. We then moved to working in the middle, the so-called "hot seat" model (see Section 5.2.5). The process involves a client working with a therapist in the middle, while the other participants sit around in a circle (in this case, on mattresses). It was explained that we used mattresses as it allowed us to be more in contact with our infantile child selves. It was not very comfortable on the mattresses as they slipped around, but at the same time it was also pleasant because lying under a blanket with two others, we cuddled. The overall atmosphere, however, was not so pleasant. I thought it resembled the trenches during the First World War because we sat in silence until someone could not stand it any longer and spoke and then they would be the one to go into the middle. The female therapist, who was a slightly authoritarian character, would smile cynically. She seemed to know which way to proceed, often confronting what the client/person in the middle was wanting to do.

When I went to the middle of the room to work on my introjects, she noticed that I was hunched in posture and keeping my body down. She got me to explore the opposite movement to what I was presenting, by asking me to stretch my body upwards. As I did this she noticed that my hands went up; so she suggested that perhaps I needed to push against something. I protested, saying that I thought my introjects didn't have much to do with this, but she explained to me quickly and persuasively that I had not been able to push against the ideas offered to me when I was younger, and so I had learned how to slouch, swallowing other people's opinions. Soon the therapist organised a few fellow male students to hold a mattress which I was supposed to then push against. I feared physical violence, looking at these men and her invitation for me to push. She comforted me, saying that this was about my need to be strong as a man and about the violence I experienced in my childhood. I was then reminded how I was beaten up several times in my childhood and how I learned to avoid confrontation. I felt like I wanted to sit down; I cried. The therapist hugged me for a moment. She then instructed me to push the mattress held by the male students. I engaged with it, feeling like I had no power. She encouraged me, asking me to add sound and to push with all the anger I held towards the boys who bullied me in childhood. I decided to push.

The therapist asked me to shout. I shouted and pushed and, after a few minutes, I noticed that I had pushed the mattress to the other side of the room. I was buzzing with pride and asked if I could push it back again to the other side of the room. I did it four times until I felt my limitation and accepted defeat. I sat back down in the group and listened to a round of feedback time in the middle. Most of it was very positive; however, at the end, a female member of the group said that she was afraid of looking at me and of the shouting. The therapist then invited this student into the middle to work on her fear of violence.

During this group, I had two opportunities to work in the middle and was coming back home fairly satisfied. When on the train, I realised that I had never loved Mariola. She was a nice woman, but I wanted someone more challenging as a girlfriend, someone who also knew how to confront me. Although my partying lifestyle continued, I noticed that I had much more energy than before, and I also attended most of my morning classes. I was happy to have so much energy, and I praised my therapy for it. Some people told me that they found me more disconnected than I was before. They told me that they thought I cared mostly about my own needs during that time, but I rejected what they said, believing that they were trying to impose their own introjects on me. I was just living and enjoying my life. After two weeks, my energy went down, and my voice changed, becoming the more familiar slightly subdued tone. I felt an emptiness when sitting in a lecture hall and couldn't understand why. The following day I skipped class and went to the students' union to work instead. It was easier, I had a task there. People asked me why had I split up with Mariola, and I noticed that I did not know what to say and eventually I articulated that we were not a good match. I was feeling pretty vulnerable. I had a sense of being robbed, like sitting in an empty home that had been plundered and as though I had lost many objects of sentimental value. Like the mining town I came from, I felt hollow underneath and on the verge of collapse. This state lasted for another week. Then I got excited. My next gestalt weekend was coming soon, and I hoped to address my low mood there.

5.1.3 Personal reflection

On writing this case study, I notice I can still feel hurt by my old psychotherapist. I can feel the amount of anger and grief over loss of time and trust spreading over my body. The earlier example verges on being emotionally, physically, and financially abusive, and I will analyse various elements of this practice later. There were two outcomes to this therapy. Firstly, I found myself depressed and ashamed following the high once the group experience was over and unable to build relationships, as shown in the example. Second, I had and still have a great deal of fear to overcome before trusting a psychotherapist.

The years following my training were years of quiet depression. I could not engage in long-term relationships as I often sought domination and feared submission. I lived with a sense of shame that there was much I needed to work on in therapy to have a good life, and I also had a feeling of not being entitled to strive for success and personal satisfaction. Now I work with clients who experienced similar treatment in Poland; they often start the therapy to improve themselves and expect me to be authoritarian and confident. This kind of hegemonic masculinity is what I expected of myself too, after finishing that particular training. I discuss this more in Chapter 4.

When I moved to London a few years after the group experience, I approached two psychotherapists, neither of whom I thought was "good enough", or perhaps even "cocky enough" to work with me. Finally, I settled for a well-established practitioner who was able to work with my fear and my criticism towards her. This was the place where I was able to build trust and finally voiced not only my anger, but also my sadness and grief towards my previous trainers and therapists. I believe that these feelings, along with my need to reflect on and come to terms with the abuse, was a driving factor in writing this chapter.

At present, I quite often find myself attacking a therapist or trainer during the initial stages of groups or individual therapy that I attend. I demand their emotional and authentic presence in the room. I would like them to prove they are with me, in a fully intersubjective way, so that not only can they have an impact on me, but I can also have an impact on them. I want them to show me they understand how my story is inevitably intertwined with their story and that they are ready to explore their "shadow" (the often repressed dark part of ourselves). I needed to see all of that to find trust.

Discovering relational gestalt built on intersubjectivity was, for me, a breath of fresh air and a theoretical support which enabled me to see, name, and deal with my abuse. However, it became another church I started to believe in. I became a missionary of this approach, watching for the "devil" in any example of non-relational work. Many, even well-intentioned psychotherapists were not able to meet my expectations, as in my body I reacted strongly to each of their words that did not fit with the relational approach. I believe that I still have these reactions, though perhaps not as strongly as before. Next I discuss an example showing how a relational approach works in practice.

This example is based on my own therapeutic work with a client whose anonymity has been preserved by fictionalising his personal details and adding elements of my own life. His emotional process was similar to mine and included fear, aggression, and building intimacy; thus, I replaced some of the content of his disclosures by inserting details from my own childhood such as: growing up on a violent estate; parents whom I felt did not have time for me; and living in a block of flats.

5.1.4 Example 2: embodied relational gestalt

I am facilitating a body therapy weekend with students of psychotherapy. I plan it to be a mixture of body experiences and personal development work. I am usually careful when offering personal development work in a group setting as students may compare themselves and feel the work they do is not so good. This time, I decided to make an exception as I wanted students who have not worked with body therapists to see how it operates. First, I invite them to move around the room, breathe, and become more aware of what they feel in their bodies and how they hold their bodies. Later I ask them to feel, through their bodies, the other people around them. We stand in the middle of the room in different constellations, playing with metaphors of what it means to have someone behind one's back or to be able to lean on someone. We start from working on sensations in our hands. When I believe they have increased their sense of touch, I ask them to shake hands with each other to notice the difference when shaking hands with each person they meet.

When we work therapeutically, I do not invite them to the middle, but work to pay attention to where they position themselves in the room. For me, it is equally interesting what happened in their childhood and how it is affecting how they are in the group now. A man tells me that he felt frightened shaking hands with other men. I invite him to shake hands with me very slowly (see Figure 5.2).

He is not able to look at me and so, paying attention to what I sensed in my body, I share. My stomach feels tense and I feel like I want to hunch and hide myself. The man then also admits that he felt something similar and discloses that this reminds him of being brought up on a violent estate where kids fought. I am listening, looking at him with a soft and moved gaze; other people in the group are silent. There is an atmosphere of care for that individual. He carries on telling us how his parents did not have time for him and would send him downstairs to play with other boys who bullied him. After a while I notice him looking at me, so I take it as a sign that he is able to carry on and have more space for my presence. Next, I notice he has hunched shoulders and ask how would he feel experimenting with switching the position. He wants to try; so he moves his chest forward

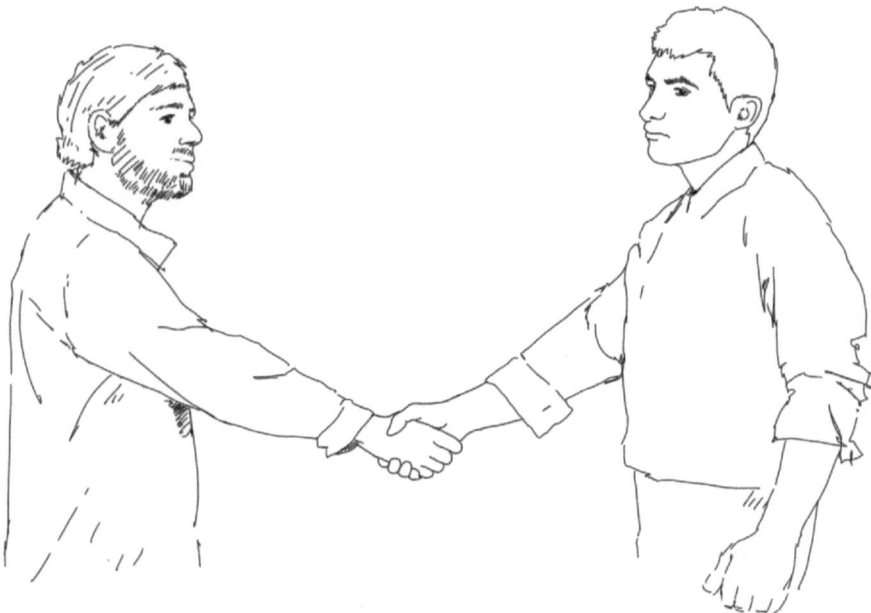

Figure 5.2 Shaking hands experiment: fear and closeness
Source: Anna Taterka (2017i).

and looks at me with very cold and angry eyes. In the first moment I am frozen, and then I decide to disclose my experiences saying:

– When you look at me I start feeling afraid of you.

– [He smiles] Indeed, I now feel angry and very confident; I feel like bullying others.

– If you were to bully me, what would you do or say?

– I could push you, or I would tell you that you are not good enough and turn around ... this is how I felt all my childhood – not good enough to be with, very lonely ... even now I often feel it with my partner. I feel so scared that I would like to push her.

– You are afraid not only of being rejected, but also of being shamed for being not good enough ...?

– Yes, that I am not strong enough ... but also not good enough to be with [he cries] ... I never understood why my parents wanted me to be out of our home that much. I thought I was a burden. They did not want me at home, and other kids did not want me outside; sometimes I was hiding in the corridor of my block.

– Do you feel there are people in this group who might like to be close to you?

– [He weeps] Yes, this is so beautiful to feel it. There are two people who I trust that they like me [he looks at them, very moved ...].

5.1.5 Analysing the journey

The earlier section was an example of relational psychotherapeutic work. It shows the relational way of working in which therapists are actively connected to their clients and share their own vulnerability in the process of attending to changing relationships within the room. That way builds the sense of belonging and attachment through vulnerability that offers a solid basis for addressing relational difficulties outside of the therapeutic room.

In this section, I will elaborate on my journey by comparing the two examples earlier. The first is the type of psychotherapy I experienced as an adolescent and during my training in Poland. Although facilitators of this approach called it gestalt therapy, it does not fit theoretically within gestalt therapy (see Section 5.2). It is fair to say that the first model is inspired by gestalt therapy and bioenergetics. The second model, Embodied Relational gestalt therapy, I learned from various sources, of which four seem to be most influential:

- My individual psychotherapy with Lesley between 2006 and 2010
- Training at Gestalt Therapy in London 2006 to 2011
- Embodied Gestalt Therapy training with Michael Clemmens in 2010
- Various trainings with Lynne Jacobs and Gary Yontef from the Pacific Gestalt Institute from 2011 onwards.

The comparison of the two examples will be based on the "hermeneutic circle" (see Section 7.5), understood as moving from particular to general and back, will include an analysis of relational dynamics, gestalt body therapy, and culture.

The Bioenergetics and gestalt-inspired body therapy accentuates self-sufficiency and independence. The assumption is that through following one's feelings and the needs implicated by them, clients would be able to self-regulate. If only we get what we need, we will be satisfied and change. My training in Poland included studying the inventors of bioenergetics: Wilhelm Reich (Reich and Carfagno, 1980) and Alexander Lowen (1994). The lack of translation of gestalt literature into Polish created a theoretical vacuum which has been filled by competitive body theories, including bioenergetics, which were integrated into the wider gestalt framework. Until now, students have learnt a therapeutic model derived from "bioenergetics body structure diagnosis" (Johnson, 1994; Lowen, 1994), whilst "embodied contact diagnosis", as outlined in Perls Hefferline and Goodman (2003), has only recently been explored. Although the trainers using that model have trained hundreds of gestalt therapists in Poland, this model has never been described and theorised; hence, they have limited any opportunity for theoretical dialogue. I chose to name this model bioenergetic gestalt to underlie its bioenergetic foundation; some writers call this model individualistic (Wheeler, 1997).

The other, "relational model" (Hycner and Jacobs, 1995), focused on how we participate in relationships around us. In line with key texts in gestalt therapy, this model accentuates contact as "the simplest and first reality [. . .] at the boundary between the organism and its environment" (Perls and Wysong, 1992, p. 1). According to Jacobs, relational gestalt therapy is based on four assumptions:

1. Relationality is irreducible [. . .]
2. We are more alike than not [. . .]
3. While our commonalities make connection possible, our individuality makes connecting interesting [. . .]
4. Our sense of self, including such dimensions as a sense of agency, emotional capacities, individuation and differentiation, and capacity for intimacy are contingent, dependent on our developmental and our immediate emotional contexts

(2009, pp. 44–47)

These four assumptions show the interdependency of human beings and fit with agential realism, providing ontological support for this research (see Chapter 6). The bioenergetic gestalt I was initially trained in is grounded in a positivistic, mechanistic view of a single person's development. The two models are therefore based on different philosophical assumptions that inform how they define emotional wellbeing and the process of change in psychotherapy.

Bioenergetics, or more precisely bioenergetic analysis or character analysis, is a type of psychotherapy originally developed by Wilhelm Reich between 1925 and 1935 (Ollendorff Reich, 1969). Focusing on his clients' non-verbal expressions of resistance towards change, he observed embodied patterns which created a character, and which could be both observed externally as well as felt through an analyst's resonance (Sletvold, 2014, pp. 24–25). The concept of character structure was developed further by his student Alexander Lowen, a co-founder of the International Institute for Bioenergetic Analysis in New York City. Lowen (1994) describes this structure as "character body armour", an armour of early life experiences and traumas that becomes embodied.

Although in his theory and practice Reich provided elements of a relational approach (Sletvold, 2014, pp. 26–27; Totton, 1998, pp. 187–194), he also used individualistic assumptions such as positioning the needs of an individual in opposition to the needs of the outer world or confronting a client's character structures as if they were individual but not co-created. The elements of the individualistic approach are presented in the Section 5.1.2 where I start believing that I need to compete for my needs in my private life, or when the therapist consistently ignores my wishes to stop the work. Critiquing the bioenergetic approach, Shapiro questions the authenticity of emotions expressed in discharging bioenergetic work:

Putting your face or your body into certain positions or configurations triggers certain emotions. The bioenergetics therapies I have seen mistake these created emotions for the release of real pent-up emotions. Their own impact in generating these emotions is not routinely explored. So, although the patient is seen as a body and a mind, the patient is a reactive object, a body that is being pushed to have a certain experience, not a body that is moving itself.

(1996, p. 310)

Analysing the shifts and a broad range of emotions during my work with the mattress, it is possible to infer that at the beginning of the group session, the therapist was guiding me into a series of *positions* to *trigger emotions*. "If therapists want to have a client hit a pillow, she or he is relatively likely to be successful", write Staemmler and Staemmler (2009, p. 70). The bioenergetic belief that emotional wellbeing comes through the expression of *pent-up emotions* was present in my early training with gestalt therapy theory in Poland. A gestalt cycle of experience (Zinker, 1977) which shows how human experiences go through cycles from relaxation through sensation, awareness, mobilisation, contact, satisfaction to withdrawal was merged with bioenergetics to create an experiment. In the imposed structure of this experiment, my subdued voice and phlegm led to an awareness of my need, mobilisation to work, contact with the mattress, the satisfaction of releasing emotions, through to my withdrawal under my blanket. The role of the therapist was to provide necessary support in each of these moments. In theory, the client should naturally move on along the cycle of experience; hence, the therapist's reaction and explanation when I felt like withdrawing from this task were aimed at motivating me to complete this cycle. Although in gestalt therapy the role of the therapist is to raise awareness (Yontef, 1993) and to support clients to be truthful to who they are (Beisser, 1970), the therapist in this case clearly had an agenda of changing me or even pushing me through change. This is an I-It, not I-Thou attitude (Buber, 2004), meaning that the therapist treats me as an object that needs to be changed, rather than a person to be met. The lack of empathy and sensitivity from the therapist may suggest aggressive behaviour or even abuse, and it certainly was experienced as such. At the end of this process, I felt misunderstood in my life and found myself looking forward to the next group. By not paying enough attention to real relationships within the group, I had a sense that there was a better world in the group and that, in real life, people were not good enough. This split was not only part of my psychological difficulty at that time, but it also turned me into some sort of therapy junkie who looks forward to the next group more than meeting his own friends.

The second example (Section 5.1.3) describes an embodied relational way of working. This model brings awareness of the relational dynamics and embodied resonance. As a group therapist in the second example, I keep returning to my embodied sensations and find ways to articulate them to the client and the group. The assumption of field theory is that the therapist's body enters the field of the client's, and hence can resonate with some of the client's emotions and body sensations. By studying the mutual impact on each other, a therapist invites a client into an honest and open relationship in which both are affecting and learning from each other. Gestalt therapists applying this model follow a cycle of embodied relational dialogue, outlined by Clemmens as:

- **Embodiment** is the sensate experience of my body/self in relation to others and the world around me
- **Attunement** is opening or reaching out with my senses to whatever "echoes" or shifts in the field (within us and our client)
- **Resonance** is the skill of noticing and amplifying my sensate response to the other person
- **Articulation** is the process of making known either to ourself or the client the experienced embodied shifts in current field circumstances.

(2012, pp. 41–43)

The embodiment is affected by previous preparation and the creation of conditions necessary for feeling embodied. The invitation at the beginning of my group (Section 5.1.3) was for the group to increase their awareness of how they held their hands and their awareness of how they breathed and sensed themselves. I moved into attunement when I invited them to notice other people through their bodies and later, when they were shaking hands, I asked them to pay attention to how they resonated with each person differently. Examples of articulation are shown when dialoguing with a member of the group.

Finally, embodied relational gestalt is based on strong ethics towards the other human being, accentuating a relational approach (Buber, 2004), empathy (Staemmler, 2012a), compassion, and self-compassion (Staemmler, 2012b).

Embodied relational gestalt begins with the assumption that our body is constantly shaped by our environment. Moment by moment, we respond to changing situations through adjustments in our body; how we look, touch, do not touch, hold our bodies, and breathe is always in relation to others. Recent neuropsychological research studies confirm this hypothesis, showing how bodily connected we are to other people (Siegel, 2010). Disconnection, therefore, is not a starting point of a relationship, but a result of aware or unaware action on our side and a denial of the importance of belonging. Thus, what kind of environment shapes a therapist to be, as in the first example, non-empathic and judgemental?

When it comes to culture, the relational attitude in psychotherapy is based on collective values. Similar values were forced upon Polish citizens both by communism and by the Catholic culture. Ten years after differentiating from communistic collectivism and in the times when the Catholic Church dominated Polish politics, people in Poland were hungry for individualism. Catholic values of sacrifice, devotion to God, and family and to the church were deeply introjected, and Polish gestalt therapy wanted to be an alternative. Even now, the so-called gestalt prayer is often quoted on the websites of many Polish psychotherapists:

I do my thing and you do your thing.
I am not in this world to live up to your expectations,

And you are not in this world to live up to mine.
You are you, and I am I,
and if by chance we find each other, it's beautiful.
If not, it can't be helped.

(Perls, 1969, cover)

Although this text has several relational editions (see Crocker, 1999, p. 275; Tubbs, 1972, pp. 77–79), some psychotherapists quote the original text that accentuates differentiation, lack of sensitivity towards the needs of others, and indifference if they are gone. As the communist regime was promoting the development of collectivist rather than individualist values, ignorance towards the collectivist nature of group process (see Section 5.2.4) in the therapy room could have also been a political rebellion. Less than ten years before that group session was held, Poland had differentiated from communism. At that time, there was a strong anti-communism, anti-collectivist attitude in Polish politics and society. Although some psychotherapists like to believe that what they do is above culture, psychotherapy has always been not only dependent on, but even in service of culture. This has been one of the major motivations in the writing of this book and in analysing cultural assumptions embedded in practice. Some examples of using psychotherapy to support homophobia are shown in Chapter 4. On the other hand, embodied relational gestalt is criticised for having a white, middle-class focus and attitude (Philippson, 2010). This way of relating requires a safety net, which is mainly affordable by white, rich, or middle-class members of European and American societies, while people struggling for money, freedom or even life, may have to be resigned to more competitive actions. In that case, the difference in the approaches may be related to an East and West divide between Poland and Western Europe.

The cultural and clinical analysis of this situation here is not exhaustive. This theoretical analysis shows the split between the two approaches and notes the bioenergetic roots of some of the Polish gestalt. In the next section, I look more critically at the theoretical ambivalences in gestalt therapy, which have led to the split presented in this chapter.

5.2 Gestalt therapy between individualism and intersubjectivity

In discussions with my international colleagues, I realise that similar bioenergetic gestalt practices are as old as gestalt therapy, take place all over the world, and can also occasionally appear in the work of relational gestalt therapists. The popularity of practitioners applying bioenergetic gestalt is gained through the use of spectacular short-term interventions creating quick changes and releases, which in the longer term possibly lead to low mood, and/or a sense of failure or resentment towards psychotherapy, as in the first example (Section 5.1.2). The first accounts of the type of work I have been describing are reported on by Frederick Perls' clients. Perls would organise large workshops in which he would present a new, efficient way of working with clients. The opinions of those clients about the ongoing results of these presentations are mixed. They range from those who felt they had been abused to accounts of life-changing experiences (Stevens, 2007).

Due to the recent popularity of relational approaches (Hycner and Jacobs, 1995) bioenergetic gestalt seems to have receded; however, there is still a close link between bioenergetic gestalt and gestalt therapy. In both examples of bodywork, therapists are working with polarities: each invites the client to try an opposite posture. The technique of exaggeration where the gestalt therapist invites a client to exaggerate, for example, a position, facial expression, or a movement, also appears in both examples. Similarly, both therapists would agree that contact, the main focus of gestalt therapy, will bring about change. Thus, what constitutes the difference that has created such different reactions in the two examples? In the sections that follow I attempt to answer that question, looking at theories of contact, aggression, field theory, phenomenology, group dynamics, and culture.

5.2.1 Dangerous empathy and righteous contact

Some people believe that it was Frederick Perls' war trauma that led him to devalue empathy in his practice (Bocian, 2010; Parlett, 2014; Staemmler, 2010). However, it seems that Perls has also become a scapegoat for unwanted elements of gestalt therapy that many of us still perform. Although he was confrontational and ambivalent in his own theory and practice, he was also warm and appreciated by some of his clients (Stevens, 2007). My experience is that most therapists integrate elements of relational and individualistic assumptions in a similar way as we may be ethically divided between collectivism and individualism, or philosophically divided between objectivism and intersubjectivity. Frequently, I have found myself "knowing" what is best for my client. I may believe that a client, or even *my* client, would benefit from a particular kind of contact or "intervention". When I am stuck, emotionally fragile, unsupported, or otherwise unavailable, I tend to limit my horizon and seem unable to see the whole diversity of options. At those times, bioenergetic gestalt is an easy resource to draw from.

Perls viewed empathy with suspicion. Quite often he did not differentiate between empathy and confluence (merging with the other); hence, he pathologised both types of contact (Perls, 1978). In a world where attunement is not permitted, people are encouraged to attend only to their needs. Although this seems to be underpinned by capitalism, also known as economic liberalism, in which decisions are to be made by individuals rather than institutions or collectives (more in Section 5.2.5), it is also an attitude of many psychologists, encouraging clients to pay attention only to their needs and to assert them against the needs of others. Recently, the concept of empathy has returned to gestalt therapy (Hycner and Jacobs, 1995; Staemmler, 2012a). Although in empathy we attend to the mutual impact one has on the other, it does not need to lead to confluence. In confluence, the "I" is diminished, while in empathy, "I" is met with "Thou". Empathy thus enables contact even if sometimes it may lead to confluence.

Imported and modified from psychoanalysis, the concept of "interruptions" of contact has also changed in recent years, inviting practitioners to be more accepting of various contact styles they may undertake. Initially Perls, Hefferline, and Goodman (2003) listed these interruptions as: projection, retroflection, introjection, egotism, and confluence, and Polster and Polster (1973) later added deflection. Each was supposed to contaminate clear contact, which was a sign of emotional wellbeing. This theory implied that there is a model of "healthy contact" that we should aspire to and that we should drop our contact interruptions to reach that state. More modern theories on this phenomenon advocate for calling them "contact modifications" (Wheeler, 1991) or "contact styles" (Joyce and Sills, 2009). This move changes the binarity of contact (on or off) into a spectrum of contacts with various shapes and forms. This non-pathologising attitude offers the opportunity to increase equality in the therapeutic room.

The increase in intersubjectivity in gestalt therapy led to a more holistic view of human development and increased equality between therapists and clients. The authoritarian position of the therapist, as in the first example (Section 5.1.2), allows therapists to tell clients how they should modify contact and lead their clients to what they believe to be more *real* contact. In that example, after diagnosing my introjects, the therapist supported me to leave them behind, to engage with "real" contact. Embodied Relational Gestalt therapists see the modifications to contact not as interruptions, but as if they were steps on a scale. For example, introjection, a habitual way of taking on other peoples' opinions, has been located on the other part of the axis from rejection. However, there is no right or wrong about choosing any of the contact styles as, for example, everyone who was ever employed knows that sometimes being able to *swallow* what a boss has said and move on can make life much easier. The therapist may raise awareness if the client gets habitually stuck or experiences *enduring relational themes* (Jacobs, 2011, 2017), a familiar pattern of behaviour reactivated and repeated in relationships. In this approach, therapists invite clients to experiment with various possibilities to discover how they may work with them, rather than offering a better alternative, as my initial therapist did in the first example (Section 5.1.2).

Gestalt's paradoxical theory of change (Beisser, 1970) supports the embodied relational way of working. The paradox of change, according to Beisser (1970), lies in the fact that in trying to change ourselves we usually fail. However, when we attend to who we are with awareness, then change occurs naturally. This difference is visible in the two autoethnographic examples. In the first one, a client is made to believe that the way he behaves in the world is wrong and needs to be adjusted, while in the second example (Section 5.1.4), the therapist guides the client through various ways he operates in the world, while raising awareness of the relational dynamics. Although awareness is believed to be the main goal of gestalt therapy (Perls, Hefferline and Goodman, 2003; Yontef, 1993), there is some recent debate that awareness may not be enough to support our clients in various moments of crisis (see Taylor, 2014; Philippson, 2014a). Again, this contradiction exemplifies a struggle to integrate various philosophical paradigms within gestalt therapy (see Chapter 6).

5.2.2 Gestalt and anger

Gestalt therapy described aggression as a positive replacement for the "psycho-analytic death instinct" (Perls and Wysong, 1992). The concept that aggression is a force leading to deconstruction and hence leads to a new quality of relationship was present in Perls' early writing (Perls, Hefferline and Goodman, 2003; Perls and Wysong, 1992). What he called dental aggression was a concept explaining human development through the function of teeth. Although it is hard to imagine the interpretive value of this metaphor, it was also applied to ideas and emotions. We want to bite, chew and decide what we want to swallow and what we would like to spit out. In the main gestalt textbook authored by Perls, Hefferline, and Goodman, this is not an individualistic process: "An emotion is the integrative awareness of a relation between the organism and environment" (2003, p. 407). However, Perls also often presented anger as individualistic, related to the expression of one's own pent-up emotions. He actively encouraged people to vent their aggression, let themselves go, or even to show a violent temper (Perls and Wysong, 1992, pp. 245–262). This does not seem to give much consideration to the other person in the relationship or indeed explain how to apply aggression in close relationships. It also reinforces the dominance of hegemonic, dominant, masculine aggressiveness as a way of interpersonal relating. While addressing difficulties leads to a *mutual advantage, venting* one's anger does not bring *the integrative awareness of a relation.*

Critiquing the cathartic practice so often present in gestalt therapy practice, Staemmler and Staemmler (2009) use a model of a hydraulic container to show how aggression is understood within the bioenergetic gestalt model. Cathartic expression of anger in the group was supposed to be a safety valve allowing the removal of the excess. Although this practice was meant to make us more able to be intimate, my experience was contradictory to that theory. Analysing the research, Staemmler and Staemmler arrive at the same conclusion:

> [T]he activity that is expected to have a "cleansing" (=cathartic) effect does not lead to the desired result – to the contrary: it boosts the person's aggressiveness in spite of her opposite expectation, i.e. against the placebo-effect, which suggests a high effect size.
>
> (2009, p. 72)

Cathartic anger could indeed lead to the avoidance of subtle and vulnerable feelings, as happened in the first example (Section 5.1.2) under the cover of creating healthy psychological wellbeing. An example of similar work done in a relational way is presented by Seidler (1997, pp. 115–116), where the author works with a boy who brought anger from school. In his example, the boy uses cushions to express his feelings, but does not throw them, shout at them, and symbolically annihilate them. He relates to them as if they were people and learns about the various perspectives from sitting in different positions.

5.2.3 Objectivistic misunderstanding of phenomenology

Husserl (1960) seemed to be ambivalent in his methodology. Although he made references to positivistic thinking, he also never believed in objectivity being achievable. His idea of *epoché* may suggest that he wanted researchers to suspend their beliefs completely to experience the thing-in-itself; in fact, he used phrases such as *objectivating acts* and the *nature of things* (Husserl and Kersten, 1983). At the same time, he was intersubjective:

> We must discover in what intentionalities, syntheses, motivations, the sense "other ego" becomes fashioned in me and, under the title, harmonious experience of someone else, becomes verified as existing and even as itself there in its own manner.
>
> (Husserl, 1960, p. 90)

Phenomenology in gestalt therapy is similarly ambivalent. On the one hand, it is reduced to what is named in qualitative research as "descriptive phenomenology". In this model, psychotherapists or researchers are to notice their experiences while suspending their judgements and histories (Spinelli, 2005). On the other hand, phenomenologists, such as Merleau-Ponty with his concept of interconnectedness through the flesh-of-the-world (Carman, 1999; Merleau-Ponty and Lefort, 1968) and Gadamer (2012), advocate for judgements to be dialogued and incorporated but not suspended. In a similar fashion, bioenergetically inspired early gestalt body therapists ignored the relational power dynamics evidenced by the confrontational style of the therapist in the first example (Section 5.1.2) and their focus on individual emotions. The New Materialism offers an integration in support of late Merleau-Ponty and Lefort (1968) that accentuates interconnection rather than objectivistic detachments. There, emotions are not located solely within the individual experiencing them:

> So emotions are not simply something "I" or "we" have. Rather, it is through emotions, or how we respond to objects and others, that surfaces or boundaries are made: the "I" and the "we" are shaped by, and even take the shape of, contact with others.
>
> (Ahmed, 2004, p. 10)

That way of making *boundaries* is congruent with the notion of dynamic and relational self in gestalt therapy (Perls, Hefferline and Goodman, 2003) and is crucial when it comes to the understanding of field theory and group dynamics, described in the next section.

5.2.4 Working with group dynamics

The bioenergetic gestalt therapy in Poland developed a non-relational way of working within the therapy groups. Gestalt group therapy in Poland was usually organised in blocks of five days' training and included two levels: one for beginners and

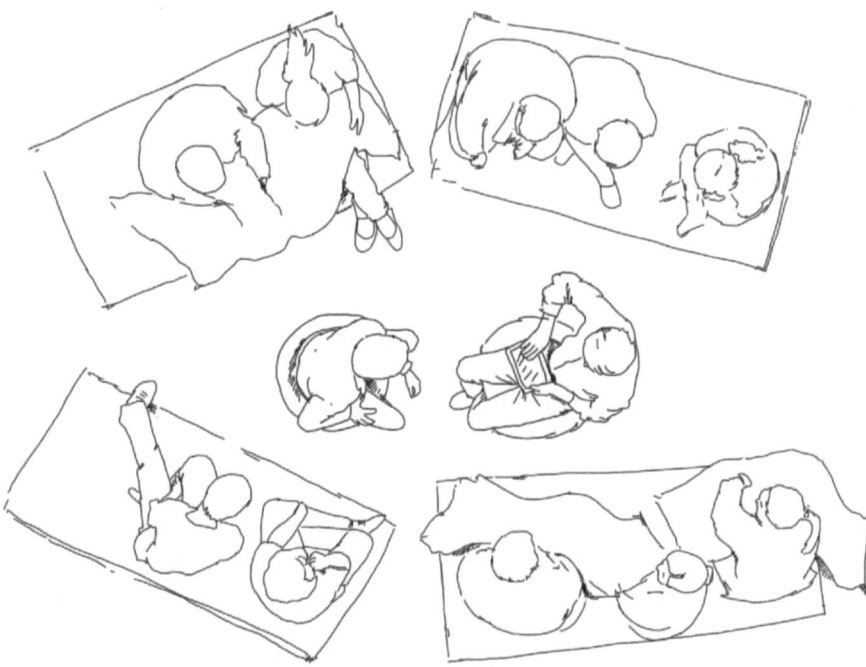

Figure 5.3 Hot seat model as used in my training in Poland

Source: Anna Taterka (2017d).

one for experienced clients. The initial training was called the Interpersonal Group and the group for experienced group attendees Personal Development Training. My critique of this structure includes the lack of an ongoing relationship between the group members and the therapist, devaluation of the interpersonal level of relating, and the emphasis on development as a personal experience. In the more advanced group they offered an almost exclusively "hot seat" model (see Figure 5.3).

The hot seat model includes two chairs in the middle of the room: one for the therapist and another for the client, while the rest of the group sit as an audience around them. Common themes in these groups are usually considered as an interesting side effect, and mutuality is not explicitly explored. A rebellion against the hot seat model in gestalt therapy came from Feder and Ronall (1980), who edited a book entitled *Beyond the Hot Seat*. This book contains one of the first formulations of gestalt group process beyond individual dynamics. In the opening article, Kepner (2008) elaborates on various group process dynamics and introduces levels of group interventions:

- Intrapersonal – personal experiences not related to people in the group
- Interpersonal – relationships with other group members and with the facilitator

- Subgroup – for example, men, women, and people who do not identify in any of these categories
- Group – whole group culture.

The role of the therapist is to shift between these levels when necessary. For example, a complaint from a group member about an inability to be honest with her husband may be explored on each of these levels as:

- Intrapersonal level – what is happening in their relationship and how this may be related to the client's early life experiences
- Interpersonal level – who in this group you may not feel honest with
- Subgroup level – who also in this group feels dishonest and who feels they are honest
- Group level – how this group impacts on individuals making it hard to be honest.

In the first gestalt body therapy group (Section 5.1.2), the therapist was not interested in the intrapersonal level even though the training was called an Interpersonal Group. A female group member who reported feeling afraid after my personal work in the middle was actively discouraged from interpersonal work with me. The therapist immediately focused on her transference: it was not that she was afraid of my behaviour; rather, she was afraid of someone else who was aggressive in her life before. The second example (Section 5.1.4) shows elements of intrapersonal, interpersonal, and subgroup levels, where the client explored how he felt with two other members of the group.

Not only is little attention paid to interpersonal dynamics in the hot seat model, but they are also discounted as less important than transference-based intrapersonal work. By naming groups as for beginners, interpersonal therapists of the hot seat model devalue relationships within the group. They suggest personal development is not related to relationships in the group. I believe that this model also fulfils some of the narcissistic needs of therapists themselves. Not only do they sit in the middle with an audience around, but also the set-up does not allow the other people to participate. Hence, the only "cure" can come from the therapist. They also cannot be challenged as a person as they always treat what other members of the group say as "transference".

Furthermore, in the hot seat model, group processes are viewed as individual ones. For example, if a group member takes the role of a scapegoat, the therapist will work with that person individually, accentuating their predispositions to take this role. In contrast, field theory emphasises awareness of the conditions necessary for this role to occur (Fairfield, 2004), rather than purely the individual's own dynamics. Treating scapegoating individually creates even further distance between that person and the group.

Similarly, any critique towards the group therapist is understood as transference, and hence pathologised. Group facilitators thus decline the opportunity to study their impact on the group. A detachment of this sort can fuel the disconnection that is often the very reason clients decide to join group therapy. The co-emergency, or using new materialist vocabulary, *an inter-agential becoming* (Barad, 2007), is not allowed in the hot seat transference model since all relationships are considered to be historical. On the other hand, radical field theorists would question whether the personal level is even possible. Since everything in any group is of-the-field (Fairfield, 2004; Hodges, 2003), the group impacts not only on how we present our issues, but also on what we choose to disclose. Radical field theorists and relational therapists would refrain from using the term "personal development". Further analysis of the way the field impacts on individual experiences requires an elaboration of cultures that create experiences. The following section compares these examples referring to capitalism and gender.

5.2.5 Collective gestalts: individualism and capitalism

Earlier, I analysed how Catholicism and communism, so embedded in Polish culture, had influenced the popularity of bioenergetic gestalt in Poland. In this section, I will look at practices that led to an individualistic approach in gestalt therapy as developed in the capitalistic culture.

The first settlers in the USA had to be self-reliant and self-sufficient. Although some, often religious, community members settled together and supported one another, the myth of the lone cowboy impacted not only American films and dreams, but also psychology and economics. Capitalist society is organised around individuals accentuating their own individual capacities rather than the collective support they receive (Wheeler, 1997). Emotional health is understood as independence and a lack of needs. Whilst working in mental health supported housing projects in East London, a place considered to be one of the most diverse places in the UK, I realised how European individualism is projected on what is considered to be emotional health, for example: the provision of only one-bedroom flats to people suffering mental distress does not fit with collective thinking and understanding of health. In this scenario, separation is a sign of emotional wellbeing. Russia is the biggest critic of Western values and sees our individualism as a reason why so many people cannot sustain relationships in our societies (McElroy, 2013). Capitalism is based on individualism. It is built on individualistic thinking and further perpetuates it. The collective lack of empathy towards other people and the environment is a feature of capitalism that has only recently started to be recognised or addressed, for example, through new materialism (Barad, 2011; Braidotti, 2013).

Individualism has led to the growth of a narcissistic culture governed by dualities, of which the biggest is success or failure. The righteous contact I describe in Section 5.2.1 is an example of that, but in psychology there is an even bigger duality: that of maturity versus childishness. The aim of therapy is believed to be maturation, often understood as a lack of relational needs and emotional reactivity. This theory is based on shame towards one's sensitivity, a fixed image of how one should be and on the destruction of relationships. It is based on a psychological belief which truly supports the current socio-economic climate and turns psycho-therapists into perpetrators of symbolic violence (Bourdieu, 1990a). Bourdieu's concern was that certain socialisations could lead people towards harmful practices. Psychotherapy, which initially critiqued this culture (for example, Freud's view on sexuality), is now reinforcing the values of a neoliberal society built on Christianity. The way that gestalt psychotherapists now focus on individual feelings and solutions is a product of capitalism (Bednarek, 2018), a system we used to contest. This way of thinking is also congruent with and supporting of hegemonic masculinity.

5.2.6 Collective gestalt of gender

What was the gender dynamic between a young Polish man and an older female Polish therapist? Brothers (2017, p. 420) suggests that the relational way of working would have been more popular if the psychotherapy founders were female, but I think she misses the hegemonic impact of the environmental conditions. In my early training, the therapist's ideas about manhood and suggestions to "man up" were left unexamined in terms of her position as a woman and her relationship with men. Was it her reprisal for how women were treated in Polish society, or perhaps an internalised oppression of clearly defined and thus rigidified genders, which the therapist encouraged me to perform?

Apart from the rigidity of gender roles, I believe that age also mattered. There was an atmosphere of seduction in the first example (Section 5.1.2) where I was challenged by her to be a man and prove it by being strong. I felt that I wanted to impress her and prove myself to have what I believed at that time to be my masculine power.

It took me over a decade to realise that masculinity in gestalt therapy did not mean confrontation. I remember a sense of puzzlement when, almost ten years after the first example (Section 5.1.2) took place, an experienced gestalt colleague admitted his vulnerability and fear of bringing his agenda to a large group meeting. At that time, I thought that being a man was to *push the mattress* and if you could not do it you certainly should not talk about this or feel okay about it. His reaching out for support, tears, and open vulnerability created an alternative experience to the one I described in this chapter and helped me to start deconstructing my rigid and hegemonic masculine embodiment.

5.3 Summary

Looking back at the first example (Section 5.1.2), I realise that, at that time of the training groups, I was constantly trying to rescue myself and my fragmented sense of who I thought I was. The lack of connection in my life mirrored the lack of connection in the group, where the moments of closeness were hidden under the blanket rather than openly explored. Therapy was an invitation to go even further away from current relationships into the world of the past, while real relational encounters were devalued, ignored, and silenced.

For Foucault (2003) and Protevi (2014), the body can be a place of knowledge or a target of abusive power. Institutionalisation, structures, and non-relational practices led to the body becoming abused and directed away from embodied knowledge. Similarly, in the first example (Section 5.1.2), the abused body was a negotiation between the personal situation and the collective gestalts of gender inequality, religious insecurity, capitalism, and communism. I feel sad and ambivalent looking back at that time. When empathising with that young man, I am tearful, and I am compassionate towards myself. At other times, I feel ashamed. I believe that similar feelings of ambivalence or conflict between different values or modes of doing gestalt therapy may now be starting to appear for some psychotherapists. The model and the examples presented here are very different, and I am aware that my experience from almost 15 years ago seems to be a harsh one, if not abusive. Since that time, I have seen few integrations of bioenergetic and gestalt therapy that were also relational and field-orientated. I also use elements of bioenergetic thinking in my work with clients. Nevertheless, I believe that the relational turn is a major cultural change for psychotherapy and that integration takes time. Psychotherapy integrates contradictory theories of which some are postmodern and relational. Collective gestalts and relational dynamics have a direct impact on the needs of our clients, and gestalt practitioners may integrate some intersubjective theories along with objectivistic ones; at the end of the day, gestalt therapy is a post-structuralist theory that allows contradictions.

Although the distinction between individualist and relational ways of working is necessary for an understanding of the therapeutic process, the polarisation which some relational therapists create out of it may be pedantic. Most of the psychotherapists I have observed move fluidly between the two and embody both individualistic and relational ways of working, with an understanding of the contradiction between the two. As time is not linear, I am also both these men in my embodied becoming, oscillating between relationality and an escape into a capitalist-infused illusion of individualism.

More practice-orientated articles, workshops, and presentations are required to discuss the integration of individualistic and contextual assumptions embedded in the practice of psychotherapy, psychology, and bodywork to challenge this culture and provide a dialogue, leading to further awareness of the interplay between both. Furthermore, as the training centres negotiate their own collective gestalts embedded in the culture and the politics of the system they are based in, training institutes need to offer creative ways of exploring culture, race, gender, and sexuality within their programmes.

My way of deconstructing collective gestalts embedded within our training and practices originated in my studies in philosophy. Although some training institutes do not provide philosophical training beyond the required minimum of Husserlian phenomenology, the majority of therapeutic concerns described in earlier chapters originated between various philosophical paradigms. The following chapter presents the philosophical map that underpinned both the content of the chapters and the autoethnographic methodology that I applied. It starts from a description of how I failed my entry exam for a degree in philosophy.

Chapter 6

Philosophies that inspired this book

This chapter is for those readers who would like to have a deeper understanding of the philosophies that shaped the way masculinity, sexuality, and culture are conceptualised in this book. If my research study were a car, so far you have seen it and driven it, and now you can look at the engine. Along with Chapter 7, it is a detailed elaboration of the theories underpinning the research study that led me to writing my PhD thesis and later this book. It is not necessary to be familiar with these theories in order to understand the chapters that treat on masculinity, sexuality, and culture; hence, I provide the philosophy and methodology chapters towards the end.

In this chapter, I further explain the agential realism briefly introduced before, along with the personal experiences that shaped my understanding and attitude towards the theory. Starting with a description of my failed entry examination for a degree in philosophy, I show how gestalt therapy led me to develop a field-orientated phenomenological perspective compatible with onto-epistemology described by Barad (2003, 2007; Barad, Dolphijn and van der Tuin, 2012). Furthermore, I integrate it with philosophies of Merleau-Ponty (2005), Buber (2004), and Gadamer (2012) that are considered critical to gestalt therapy (Frank, 2001; Joyce and Sills, 2009; Staemmler, 2010).

6.1 Post-communist deconstructionism

"Why do you want to study philosophy?" asked an interviewer at the access examination for the philosophy degree in Wrocław when I was 18 years old.

I was a middle-class child straight from high school and the question of what I would do after a five-year master's programme in philosophy, or more concretely the history of philosophy, had not occurred to me. Philosophy was not the passion of my heart, but at that time I did not know what was. I knew that university is something that one does after high school, a thought that I realised later in my life belongs to a class intelligentsia present in most Communist and post-communist societies. At that time, I had had therapy for two years related to my insecurities, and although I had some emotional understanding, I wanted to deepen my philosophical thinking about the world and my relation to and within it.

> "I want to understand humans," I replied.
> "Which one concretely?" answered the examiner, and the whole examination board laughed.

That was the beginning and the end of my examination, which lasted no more than five minutes. It was the first ever post-structuralist critique of my thinking that resulted in failing the entry interview, placed my faith in Katowice, not Wrocław, as a location for my studies. It was also the first time I learned how emotionally tough studying philosophy would be and how little attention the lecturers paid to the emotional impact of shame or any other feelings for that matter. The same attitude occurred at the University of Silesia in Katowice; however, I was more prepared after that painful initiation. Although this attitude could be seen as a part of masculine competitiveness that eliminates feelings through shaming, later in this chapter I elaborate on two other sources that contribute to the popularity of deconstructionism in post-communist countries: the origins of European philosophy, and the post-communist need to differentiate from collectivism.

One of the first early philosophers, Socrates, described two ways to get to know philosophy: *elenctic* and *maieutic* (Reale and Catan, 1990). While *elenctic*, also known as Socratic questioning, was the art of asking questions in a way that demonstrated inconsistencies in the interlocutor's thinking, *maieutic* was supposed to be the art of getting new knowledge from the person we converse with. Etymologically based on the Greek word "*maia*" meaning "midwife" (interestingly that was Socrates' wife's profession), it was supposed to be a gentle process of excavating internal knowledge through the dialogue. Unfortunately, Socrates and Plato either did not elaborate on this method in their lifetime or hid it only for special students; thus, we do not have any written material about how to apply this method.

I think this is what contributed to the slightly aggressive and polemical attitude of my university lecturers and the success of deconstructionism in post-communist societies. In 1997, Derrida received an honorary doctorate from the same university I joined only a year later to study philosophy. The need to rebel against the restricting notions of realism or, more precisely, socio-realism and collectivism is also strongly felt, and the rebuff I got at the five-minute interview was also part of this culture.

After the Second World War, there was a wave of surrealism and abstraction that was trying to deal with the war trauma and the inability to contain the reality that was so monstrous. At that time, Picasso was invited to Poland and celebrated for his abstract art; however, from the end of Stalinism in 1957, the attitude changed. The only art that was accepted was that which was understandable to the masses and showing the achievement of a simple man. Similarly, in research and philosophy, what was real and led to the emancipation of the masses or a critique of the rich was allowed. Marxism and realism were the right theories to practise, while social constructivism and relativism were seen as too "Western" and based on individualistic needs (subjective). The research studies that had in mind the benefit of the masses and the collective were officially accepted and sponsored. It was not just the matter of subsidies; there was a real fear of how bad opinion in the Communist party could lead to imprisonment or have a long-lasting effect on your career. This is why, with the collapse of the Iron Curtain, there was a surge in the relativistic research that deconstructed structures and prioritised singularity (similarly to the impact of individualism on the application of gestalt therapy in Poland described in Chapter 5).

> Like all theories, deconstruction was a message in a bottle. It floated off, generously but unpredictably [. . .]. [T]he fascination in Poland, in the Czech Republic, and in Hungary with deconstruction – exemplified by the honorary doctorate given to Derrida in 1997 by the University of Silesia [. . .] – obviously can't be understood by assuming that post-structuralism's intervention in the discourse of the Socialist Bloc functioned in the same way as it did in France, Britain, or the USA.
>
> (Terdiman, 2009, p. 198)

The impact on me as a student was strong. After several years of ongoing deconstruction of my thoughts and ideas, I felt quite depressed and humiliated. I struggled to attend my university. In my second year, I started to study at a second faculty, Social Work, and so I had permission to miss some, but not all, of my classes. In Chapter 5, I describe further how, as an outcome of this, I returned to gestalt therapy, seduced by the charisma of some of the trainers. Eventually, at my university, I decided also to follow gestalt therapy and, in 2004, I graduated with a thesis exploring the philosophical underpinnings of gestalt therapy: the phenomenology of Husserl and Merleau-Ponty, and the existentialism of Sartre and Buber. Through my experiences at the university, I learned to listen to my body and focus on the feelings and embodiment that underpin intellectual debates. It was a deflection from these debates into an area in which I felt not only confident, but also some sense of superiority. Being afraid of further humiliation, I learned to hide from intellectual debates inside and look at the reasons why some areas created a number of emotions and a structure of power dynamics that underpinned this exchange. That was a tiring and isolating job and I can only imagine how much fear I had at that time to keep it as a default. Max Scheler (2017) was one of the first philosophers to wonder whether the psychoanalysis of a situation undermines the philosophical argument, and found that there is no ground to discredit a thought on the basis of the speaker's latent emotional motives. Although the superiority that this strategy offered me appeared similar to the one my entry examination interviewers had, it was a good enough solution to deal with the amount of shame and competitiveness that I felt as a student of philosophy.

Gestalt therapy in Poland at that time was also taught in a shaming way (see Chapter 5). The post-communist need for separation from the collective and rebellion over the structured schooling system of the Communist years led to indi-vidualism and an attack on thinking. During my gestalt training in Poland, I felt shamed for being too intellectual, giving too little attention to my intuitive bodily reactions and feelings. Amongst the most common reactions of shame are blushing, cringing, sinking feeling, low speech, lack of eye contact, restrained spontaneity, freezing, low esteem, feeling ridiculous, discomfort, dropping of the head, and a contraction and withdrawal of the body, and discouragement (see Kaufman, 1980; Lee, 1995; Resnick, 1997; Wheeler, 1997). I experienced most of these reactions, along with a feeling that there was something inherently wrong with me, as I could not relate to people in an emotional way, but only upset them through my intellectu-alisations, while in my philosophy studies I could not fully relate intellectually and was too sensitive. I remember my therapists and other group participants instructing me frequently: "No, Adam, this is a thought; what do you feel?" until I learned to speak in a purely phenomenological way about my sensations, hiding my thoughts and judgements as well as I could. It was only later in my development as a gestalt therapist that I learned about the relational approach and about gestalt therapists who include philosophy and believe that each thought has many feelings in it. Care-ful listening to clients or friends who talk intellectually can unravel a large variety of feelings. That was the beginning of a true integration and the development of my style as a psychotherapist, a trainer, and a great relief to my shame.

Around the same time, in my mid and late 20s, I was taught by a tutor at the Gestalt Centre in London who enlightened me that people are not logical beings and opened me up to the possibility of seeing ourselves as contextual (field depen-dent) and fractured (multiple selves). This truly post-structuralist lesson in the self as fractured, multiple, and non-essentialist was reinforced by my doctoral aca-demic supervisors at the University of Brighton who introduced me to Foucault, Deleuze, Guattari, and Barad, whom I quote frequently in this book.

In the construction of my intellectual underpinning, I also need to credit my father who taught me about prejudices and dialogue (see Chapter 2) and the need to stay dialogic and truthful to my own values. Assuming these are dynamic and fractured, they may keep me away from the absolutism and certainty that he saw growing up in Germany in the 1930s.

All these experiences led me to look for an ontology and epistemology that are not only congruent with phenomenological attention to body and bodily sensa-tions, but also see the body as conditioned by the cultural and discursive per-spective. A theory and a way of being that embrace diversity, but do not lose the individual, see us as fractured beings, but also as responsible for our choices, dependent and free, boundary-less, and boundaried.

6.2 Agential realism: flesh-of-the-world or matter-of-perception

The first theory that I found compatible with my way of thinking and conceptu-alising research was the concept of *flesh* by Merleau-Ponty (Merleau-Ponty and Lefort, 1968), a concept that was not fully defined and elaborated. Merleau-Ponty died before publishing *The Visible and the Invisible* (1968) and was therefore not able to specify or answer questions regarding the concept. I interpret Merleau-Ponty's *flesh* as a unique connection of body, mind, and movement, always embedded in a relational, cultural, and social context. Merleau-Ponty argued that *flesh* guarantees a unique connection of ourselves with the world (invisible with visible):

> The world seen is not "in" my body, and my body is not "in" the visible world ultimately: as flesh applied to a flesh, the world neither surrounds it nor is surrounded by it.
>
> (Merleau-Ponty and Lefort, 1968, p. 138)

Flesh is not matter, but an interlinking element. In this concept, Merleau-Ponty reaches for the pre-Socratic concept of *arche* (Greek: ἀρχή), the essential interlinking element on which the world was founded (for example, water for Thales of Miletus). Merleau-Ponty accentuates the dynamic nature of *flesh*, and its inseparability of body and mind, and subject and object.

A similar, wide-reaching concept is presented by the quantum physicist Barad, who, arguing for the inseparability of subject and object (as well as body and mind), introduces the term *ethico-onto-epistemological matter* (Barad, Dolphijn and van der Tuin, 2012). While Merleau-Ponty saw *flesh* as an interlinking element, for Barad *matter* (further defined in the following section) is alive and both inseparable and separated from the observer. In her writing, she refers to another quantum physicist, Niels Bohr, and his experiments, showing the impact of direct observation on the observed phenomena (Barad, 2007; Nichol, 2005, p. 124).

Barad calls her ethico-onto-epistemology *agential* realism, a theory in which she initially agrees with Foucault on how various social practices shape matter. However, she criticises Foucault for not giving enough consideration to how matter shapes the practices: "Language matters. Discourse matters. Culture matters. There is an important sense in which the only thing that does not seem to matter anymore is matter," writes Barad (2003, p. 801). The physicist suggests abandoning representationalism in research (the focus on how matter is represented, which only reinforces the split between object and subject) and focusing instead on performativity (practice, actions). What she calls *agential intra-action* is the essence of this performativity. It is the moment of intersubjective contacting (linking subject and object), experiencing, acting, not upon something but always in conjunction with it. *Agential intra-action* is the place where we are experiencing and have response-ability towards matter. To use an example from therapeutic practice, *intra-action* is the moment of body to body contact where we feel both the connection and separation, the impact of the other person on us and our impact on them, where we do not diagnose but engage, where the politics of the situation call us to respond and where the newness happens.

There are many similarities between the *flesh* and *agential realism*. Although Merleau-Ponty did not refer to materialism, his later work aimed "to explain a generative, self-transformative, and creative materiality without relying on any metaphysical invocation of mysterious, immaterial forces or agencies" (Coole, 2010, p. 93). His concept of perception as flesh and flesh as perception (Merleau-Ponty and Lefort, 1968; Kennedy, 2013) is akin to Barad's agential matter, and last but not least, both Barad and Merleau-Ponty critique the anthropocentric attitude in which only human matter matters (Connolly, 2010, p. 178). The ethics of our response-ability in relationship with nature removes the anthropocentric belief that nature and other species are subordinate to us and invites us to consider matter as an intra-active being. Similar values are expressed by Buber (2004).

6.3 The philosophy of integration of body and mind, subject and object, and matter and form

Following the development of intersubjectivity, I see Barad's work both as a critique and an extension of the work started by Husserl and early Merleau-Ponty. She holds the deeply intersubjective belief of the inseparability and co-creation of the apparatus (of perception) and the perceived; neither of them are passive. She claims that we "enter not as fully formed, pre-existing subjects but as subjects intra-actively co-constituted through the material-discursive practices that [we] engage in" (Barad, 2007, p. 168). This is similar to the gestalt therapy concept of self as emerging from a situation (Perls, Hefferline and Goodman, 2003; Wollants, 2012). The shaming environment of my university and post-communist Poland impacted me in such a way that I was shaming towards my partner during those days (see Chapter 5). I undermined her and kept on recommending therapy, suggesting that I was much more enlightened than her because of my own experience. Nowadays, I aim to see emotions as relationally co-emergent; for example, feelings felt by a partner in a relationship are part of what is happening between people involved in this relationship and the wider field. If I feel lonely in a relationship, I wonder what this says about myself, the people around me, my wider group of friends, my past, the political situation, etc. These examples are concerning humans. However, true intersubjectivity can only happen when we include the matter that in a dialogic way will challenge the primary position of humans in a much larger universe. How does the destruction of the environment and extinctions of species impact my loneliness and how does my loneliness impact other animals and objects around me? Could there be a link?

> The tree will have a consciousness, then, similar to our own? Of that I have no experience. But do you wish, through seeming to succeed in it with yourself, once again to disintegrate that which cannot be disintegrated?
>
> (Buber, 2004, p. 15)

Husserl's focus on empathy keeps the semantics of the interaction within the anthropocentric paradigm, while Merleau-Ponty uses the word flesh, which extends to animals. Barad's choice of vocabulary is matter. She sees the world as dialoguing not only on the discursive, but also physical (for example, quantum) level, rather than only within the body or mind. If we imagine a stone, its structure is entirely dependent on the environment; the stability it receives is a matter of temperature, air, and other factors. If we change the temperature, the stone may melt or break. Furthermore, this stone is dialoguing on a molecular level with the environment (Barad, Dolphijn and van der Tuin, 2012), taking over time the qualities of air and ground it is placed on. Every interaction is unique and is indeed a dialogue. Each of these dialogues produces a new matter through its ongoing intra-actions. Although this thought may seem controversial in the field of psychotherapy based on anthropocentric humanism, Barad's idea of intra-actions corresponds to Buber's *I-Thou* dialogue which has been widely used to describe the nature of the therapeutic relationship. This quote often makes me cry: ". . . if I have both will and grace, [. . .] in considering the tree I become bound up in relation to it. The tree is now no longer It" (Buber, 2004, p. 14). For Buber, a tree is an event that dialogues with us, an interaction where I have a possibility to be changed. His *I-Thou* combination (Buber, 2004) (a soulful relation) is applicable to the relationships both with people and nature. As does Barad, Buber proposes to overcome the split between nature and culture by redefining the matter as agential. In a critique of Foucault, Barad (2007) replaces his *discursive practices* with *material-discursive practices*, and states that every intra-action is impacted by and impacting on *material-discursive practices*. What about gestalt therapy: do we understand dialogic as materially dialogic when we speak about the embodied relational practice?

6.4 Body and matter

Merleau-Ponty defined perception as an active, embodied, relational, and creative process (Vasseleu, 1998, p. 24). Body sensations were the gateway to knowing the *flesh-of-the-world*. "Phenomenology [of Merleau-Ponty and Husserl] helps us to explore how bodies are shaped by histories, which they perform in their comportment, their posture, and their gestures" (Ahmed, 2010, p. 246). Similarly, in my research, I focus on discursive embodied sensation as a critique of the discourses that create the separation between bodily experiences (*flesh*) and their contexts (see Section 7.5). The focus on emotions and sensations of *flesh* provides a gateway between Barad's onto-epistemology and the embodied research methodology applied in this book.

In the later part of his life, Merleau-Ponty placed greater emphasis on *body schema*, to which access is required to experience the out-of-awareness (Merleau-Ponty and Lefort, 1968). The *flesh* is considered with its history (*schema*), and research and discovery are focused on the *flesh of the world*; I accentuate the "of" to show the anti-representationalism that Merleau-Ponty implied. We (*flesh, matter*) are not separated in the world, but of the world. Returning to Barad: we are both agential and discursive (see the following section).

Merleau-Ponty's (Merleau-Ponty and Lefort, 1968, Merleau-Ponty, 2005) perception was corporeal, each mental state a body phenomenon. He claimed that our perception is not a passive state or, to use more embodied language, our perceiving-body is in a constant flux of sensorimotor action. I like to use dance to illustrate how, in constant movement, I learn not only about my myself and my partner, but also about the orchestra, the dance floor, and the attitudes of other dancers and spectators. Merleau-Ponty (2005) notices that every observation of an external phenomenon brings internal resonance. Likewise, every internal phenomenon has a relationship with the outside environment. Many philosophical dichotomies, such as outside and inside, objective and subjective, body and mind, nature and culture, knower and known, are inseparable in his thinking.

Similarly, in Barad's theory, "agency is about response-ability, about the possibilities of mutual response, which is not to deny, but to attend to power imbalances" (Barad, Dolphijn and van der Tuin, 2012, p. 55). She believes that what increases objectivity is not the distance necessary in methodologies deriving from realistic traditions, but the response-ability, understood as an embodied interaction with an awareness of power dynamics. It is the mutual embodied interaction with awareness of power that makes Barad's theory so like gestalt therapy. However, what gestalt therapy does not spell out is how to attend to the power imbalances. In order to attend to power imbalances in a relational way, I will return to the philosophy of Gadamer (2012) that was already introduced in Chapter 2.

6.5 Intra-acting

Agential realism (Barad, 2007) integrates the paradox of being constructed through the encounter and having separate agency. An article on phenomenology and the new materialism explains it well:

> [The] emphasis on corporeality further dislocates agency as the property of a discrete, self-knowing subject inasmuch as the corpus is now recognized as exhibiting capacities that have significant effects on social and political situations. Thus, bodies communicate with other bodies through their gestures and conduct to arouse visceral responses and prompt forms of judgment that do not necessarily pass through conscious awareness.
>
> (Coole and Frost, 2010, p. 20)

That idea of historical necessity and agential response-ability is encapsulated by Gadamer's definition of dialogue (2012). For Gadamer, dialogue is an opportunity to realise our own prejudices by contacting the other.

The inter-acting events (for example, two people) are being constructed in this encounter. The agential differentiation between the therapist and the client (the researcher and the researched) is created through this interaction. In gestalt therapy, *self* is being created throughout each of the interactions and does not exist in separation (Perls, Hefferline and Goodman, 2003), and for Barad, "the condition of possibility for objectivity is therefore not absolute exteriority but agential separability – exteriority within phenomena" (2007, p. 184). The *material-discursive practice* that we engage with creates a sense of boundaries and separation of matter that is contextual and evolving. The emerging separation between the researcher and research is crucial for the design of this book, where each findings chapter is based on *agential separability* that is forming and evolving as the text progresses.

Although my *flesh* is inevitably informed by my past and inter-agentially dependent on my environmental circumstances, I am making choices on what matter will matter. The choice of our research subject is a deeply ethical matter:

> [W]hat we need is something like an ethico-onto-epistem-ology – an apprecia-tion of the intertwining of ethics, knowing, and being – since each intra-action matters, since the possibilities for what the world may become calls out in the pause that precedes each breath before a moment comes into being and the world is remade again, because the becoming of the world is a deeply ethical matter.
>
> (Barad, 2007, p. 185)

Since our choices are both deterministic and free, what matters is the choice we make to attend to the determinacies: the material-discursive practices that produce us. Gadamer's emphasis on attending to dialogue as a never-ending way to realise our own prejudices (horizon) (2012) has been a great inspiration for my writing and data analysis (see Section 7.5) as it encapsulates the need for an *I-Thou mattering dialogue*. Gadamer was raised in the territory that now belongs to Poland and he lived through both World Wars. His idea of dialogue is so important to me as it encapsulates my family's constant dialogues between Polish and German roots (see Chapter 2). The *I-Thou mattering dialogue* of my research is an attempt to notice the construction of matter in its deeply historic, societal, political, personal, and embodied way.

Barad's agential realism conceptualises the overarching ethico-onto-epistemology of this book and my understanding of gestalt therapy. Her research apparatus is discursive, but not sufficiently sensuously embodied. By introducing Merleau-Ponty's flesh, I illustrate the epistemological potential of the human body that is shaped by material-discursive practices. A practical way to uncover these practices lies in the idea of dialogue that brings out our own prejudices (Gadamer) in dialogue with both animate and inanimate matter (Buber; Barad).

For Merleau-Ponty, "our bodily skills and dispositions carve out a perceptual world with perspectival horizons" (Carman, 2008, p. 133). Every study of the world will always be a study of a researcher's body and its horizons. This has not only been a tool, but also a central focus of my writing. By attending to my body as intra-active (*horizontal flesh-of-the-world*), I aim to attend to culture, relationships, and philosophy through my constantly evolving embodiment, providing a unique snapshot of my sensations and their contexts. Knowledge will be created and will come out of movement and bodily interactions *of* the context of societal and relational dynamics. Agency, according to Barad, is "reconfiguring the material-discursive field of possibilities and impossibilities in the ongoing dynamics of intra-activity" (2007, p. 170). Autoethnography as a research methodology can serve this purpose well.

Chapter 7

Culture as ground; personal becoming as figure

Autoethnography and gestalt therapy

Autoethnography and gestalt therapy can form a marriage of both love and convenience. The intuitive connection between ethnographic approaches and field theory, as well as between individual stories and phenomenology, provides a basis for this relationship. The mutual appreciation lies also in the relationship to the aesthetics as both gestalt therapists and autoethnographers focus on aesthetic criteria, paying attention to their work being engaging, stimulating, gracious, and moving.

Autoethnography as a research methodology allows gestalt therapists to integrate ethnographic and phenomenological research methodologies. Whilst ethnography is designed to study the culture, phenomenology encourages the researcher to start the exploration from unique individual sensations. Gestalt therapy since its beginnings has been concerned with the organism-environment field, hence its study of the unique relationship between personal and cultural, the figure and background dynamics.

However, autoethnography also challenges and further develops gestalt therapy theory and practice. It provides a way to communicate the outcomes of the research beyond the gestalt therapy community. It also invites explicit critical examination of cultures that create embodiments, and therefore is applicable to those researchers who want to interrogate the ground through the unique study of the known figure. The figure is based on individual experiences. This book encourages the use of autoethnography in gestalt therapy that could further support master's and doctoral level research studies into culture and embodiment. Furthermore, it also aims at enriching this research methodology through bringing the psychotherapeutic and more unique gestalt perspectives on embodiment and phenomenological method to ethnography.

The research discourse in gestalt therapy in the last two decades oscillates between using approaches that demonstrate the efficiency of gestalt therapy through methodologies accepted by the American Psychological Association (Brownell, 2014), and developing a research methodology that is based on gestalt therapy values and tradition (Barber, 2006).

The first approach is fuelled by our survival anxieties. Because of limited research on the efficiency of gestalt therapy in the past, in some countries the gestalt therapy situation deteriorated. In the UK, gestaltists do not usually work in the National Health Service unless they learn, apply, or pretend that they do other psychotherapeutic methodologies, mainly CBT, systemic or psychodynamic. There is a concern that psychotherapy and counselling may be limited to a small number of methodologies in the same way that the National Institute for Health and Care Excellence decides which antidepressants will be available in the UK market (NICE, 2019). Gestalt therapists therefore need to produce substantial research that makes us visible and can convince health authorities about the usefulness of the approach.

Another strand of gestalt therapy research aims at designing the research that improves gestalt therapy using gestalt therapy methodology (e.g. Barber, 2006). The unique combination of phenomenology, field theory, and relational attitude can be adapted for rigorous research and provides insightful qualitative research studies, but these are read mainly by gestalt therapists who usually use them to improve their practice.

The aim of this book is to introduce autoethnography as valid and consistent with gestalt therapy methodology in the study of psychotherapy, and to seed some ideas from gestalt therapy amongst ethnographic researchers. Autoethnography resonates with agential realism (Barad, 2007), an onto-epistemology that fits with gestalt therapy ideas about dynamic selves, simultaneous separation, and dependency on the context (Perls, Hefferline and Goodman, 2003). The autoethnographic focus on cultures including gender, sexual orientation, ageing, class, disability, race, and ethnic diversity offers discussions that are not taking place within gestalt therapy enough (see Chapter 4).

Gestalt therapy has the potential to offer autoethnography a revised understanding of embodiment as a co-created relational dynamic of the researcher and the researched. Gestalt therapy and new materialism (Barad, 2007; Coole and Frost, 2010; Fox and Alldred, 2017) further accentuate the inevitable impact of the researcher on the subject, in fact they claim radical mutuality understood as co-emergence of the subject and the researcher. Furthermore, our strong focus on here-and-now contact as well as ethics are tools that researchers can find useful in the application of autoethnographic methodology. The focus on early developmental embodiments and movements (Frank and Barre, 2011) and interpersonal communication enhance current dimensions explored by autoethnographers, and may prove to be useful during data collection and analysis.

This chapter provides both an introduction to autoethnography as a research method for gestalt therapy and a description of the methodological considerations that I had to make when designing the research study that is presented in this book.

7.1   Introducing autoethnography as a way to study embodied sensations

Autoethnography is a research methodology that focuses on personal memory as a valid source of knowledge (Ellis, Adams and Bochner, 2010). By attending to personal memories, autoethnographers reconstruct a version of truth, which is then analysed using the ethnographic methodology. The truth is relative (Geertz, 2000), subjective, provisional, and fragmented (Grant, Short and Turner, 2013), as autoethnographers, like gestalt therapists, do not believe in truth existing independently. They treat data as social events that are situated representations (Atkinson, 1990), similar to my interest in discovering the contexts of my situatedness through represented experiences, as discussed in previous chapters. However, autoethnography is not merely a reconstruction of memory, but a method designed to challenge cultural assumptions and systemic stagnations within the field. As Grant (2019, p. 90) puts it, it requires a researcher to be "a wolf".

Autoethnography began as a reaction to the positivist and post-positivist paradigm in science where the "scholar is seen (in the credits) but not heard (in the text)" (Sparkes, 2002a, p. 213). On a more practical level, it is a way of "reflexively writing the self into and through the ethnographic text; isolating the space where memory, history, performance, and meaning intersect" (Denzin, 2013, p. 22). Whilst personal writing makes statements about memory, history, performance, and meaning, according to Jones, Adams and Ellis (2013, p. 22), autoethnography requires the research to be as follows:

1   Purposefully commenting on/critiquing of culture and cultural practices;
2   Making contributions to existing research;
3   Embracing vulnerability with purpose; and
4   Creating a reciprocal relationship with audiences in order to compel a response

Etymologically, auto-ethno-graphy refers to the old Greek words for *myself, people/culture*, and *description/analysis* (Collins English Dictionary, 2014). It is a unique and critical study of the researcher embedded in a cultural and relational context. Autoethnography offers a challenge to more traditionally understood realism as it uses constructionist or materialist-dialogic epistemology. Whilst positivist research claims that the validity of research is enhanced by a high number of cases, autoethnography focuses on individual, personal accounts, believing that they can bring deep insights into researched phenomena (Zeeman, Aranda and Grant, 2014).

Autoethnographic writing emerges from retrospective field notes (Ellis, 2004) and has been described as unofficial texts (Ellis, 1995) as it focuses on personal and often intimate reports, and does not have fixed genres. Researchers following this method use various media such as prose, poetry, performance, film, and art to create a reciprocal relationship with audiences. It is about being evocative as well as descriptive. Attention is paid, therefore, to aesthetics and to different ways of engaging readers and audiences. An autoethnographer's focus goes beyond academic papers and includes the impact their research can have on audiences, as well as its further social and political impact.

Autoethnography usually demands a "multi layered level of researcher reflexivity" (Grant, Short and Turner, 2013, p. 1) which offers a deep and critical focus on the researchers as well as on the context of the research. Reflexivity requires autoethnographers to be transparent not only with their research participants, but also with their readers and, most of all, themselves, showing their values, goals, and cultural assumptions. It is a way of showing not only *what* was discovered but also *how* it was discovered (Etherington, 2007).

Autoethnography has become more popular in psychotherapy in recent years, with some therapists writing about their own bodies in this way. The popularity of autoethnography in psychotherapy is due to the methodology, providing a means for understanding and healing (Etherington, 2003).

> Flesh to flesh methodologies stand in multi-figured contrast to fixed truth-seeking methods.
>
> (Spry, 2001, p. 727)

Explicitly embodied autoethnography focuses on various aspects of the human body and embodiment. Although all of the embodied autoethnographers state that they want to restore the connection of body and mind, some focus on illuminating this connection, some on describing their illnesses or ageing, and some on the use of the body as a means of communication through performance.

The term embodied autoethnography is usually associated with performers who choose this methodology to be able to include what is being communicated through their bodies (Spry, 2011). They treat embodiment as a valid source of knowledge and experience, which liberates knowledge and academic research from Cartesian body-mind dualism (Bartleet, 2013, pp. 452–453) and the epistemological objective/subjective split (Spry, 2001, p. 724). In performance, the embodied autoethnographer's body is both a source of data and a means for disseminating the results. As shown in the following quotation, embodied data collection is an inter-subjective process, which enables and enriches communication.

> When my body vibrates with the gravitational pull of another body's version of reality, I know that I need to release my own gravitational hold on reality and dialogically engage this other time and space [. . .] [I]t is about embodying and critically evaluating the complex impulses of communication.
>
> (Spry, 2001, p. 725)

This shows how similar is the practice of embodied autoethnographers and gestalt therapists who also need to release their *own gravitational hold* on their own reality to dialogically engage.

Other embodied autoethnographers write about concerns such as illnesses (Ettorre, 2005), trauma (Etherington, 2003), putting on weight (Stanley, 2015), and ageing (Sparkes, 2013). Here, emphasis is put on the symptoms that appear when the body sends signals which are strongly felt messages of bodily processes. They create unique diaries of difficult experiences of embodiments, describing moments which cause deep life concerns where we would prefer to detach from our bodies and stay in our minds away from sensations.

Essén and Värlande (2013) attend to how to sharpen awareness of the body and body sensations. They suggest the integration of phenomenological attention to bodily sensations along with autoethnographic methodology. For embodied auto-ethnographers and gestalt therapists, the body has the same function as a micro-scope for the microbiologist.

> [S]ensuous experience is far from isolated from history or from social or textual norms. Rather, there is a continuous movement between the social and material, between the individual and cultural, a dialectic which occurs in the flesh.
>
> (Essén and Värlander, 2013, p. 416)

It is also important to consider whether it is possible to describe the body and if so, then how. The psychoanalyst Stern (2000) claimed that the *verbal self* develops much later than our sense of embodiment; hence, it is difficult to verbalise the pre-verbal body. The academic format of a text limits embodied experiences (Essén and Värlander, 2013, p. 406). Critiquing post-structuralist and feminist approaches to the body, Stoller (1997) notices that although they liberate the body from objectivistic desensitisation, the language they use is detached and disembodied. He invites the use of metaphors, embodied, spiritual-like language as well as humility to capture what is sensuous. Similarly, Sparkes' (2002b) advice is to use poetry to capture embodiment. Sparkes' research develops a language for talking about body sensations in the moment, using poetry and drawings.

Apart from embodied autoethnography, an autophenomenographic approach provides a more advanced integration of ethnographic and phenomenological approaches. The term autophenomenography was most probably used for the first time by Gruppetta (2004) for autoethnographic research that did not focus solely on culture, but on the researcher's own topics of interest. Since that time, it has been popularised by Allen-Collinson (2011, 2013), who focused mainly on using this method in researching sporting activities. Autophenomenography allows for a more intimate interplay between embodied sensations and ethnographic research of oneself. Similar to autoethnography, it is a study of the researcher within the context of culture, politics, and relationships (Allen-Collinson, 2013). However, the difference between autoethnography and autophenomenography is significant and methodological. While autoethnography is grounded in the ethnographic tradition, autophenomenography allows integration of both phenomenological and ethnographic traditions.

My research study that provided a basis for this book freely borrowed elements from both embodied autoethnography and autophenomenography. The integration of phenomenological and ethnographic traditions in my research was facilitated by the constant focus on embodied experiences within their contexts. Collecting data, I integrated sensation-centred phenomenological interviews with field notes and used personal documents often associated with ethnography. When analysing data, I used Gadamer's *hermeneutic cycle* to enhance the relationship between sensuous experiences and culture, while the dissemination of data was inspired by creative methods embedded in autoethnographic performativity and gestalt therapy experimentation in my workshops, presentations, and this book. I will now detail my own autoethnographic methodology, and provide some practical steps for emerging gestalt autoethnographers.

7.2 Undertaking autoethnographic research in gestalt therapy

Although this process may seem traditional and is artificial, I find it useful to look at the research process as a journey from finding a research question, considering the methodology and methods, making ethical considerations, collecting data, analysing them, and disseminating. Next, I describe how to select a research question and choose a methodology. This chapter is written for gestalt therapy students who are completing their final thesis and other types of researchers within gestalt therapy writing articles or doctoral studies. Some considerations about methods, ethics, and how to work with autoethnographic data are presented in the following two sections using this book as an example.

7.2.1 Finding a research question

A research question is one that encapsulates the topic of the research study and indicates methodology. A typical autoethnographic research question will include an "I statement" often starting from the words "How do I . . .?" and refers to the study of culture. My experience is that students either go blank, or get muddled or overambitious when selecting their research question.

Considering the difficulty of juggling personal life, a job that needs to pay for the training, psychotherapeutic placement, and other demands of psychotherapy training, it is important to select a theme that does not give us more work. A useful and playful theory that I adapted from my work at a transpersonal institute suggests that we do not choose the topic, but the topic chooses us (Romanyshyn, 2007). Precisely because the passivity of the topic choosing a researcher may seem confusing for gestalt therapists (who like to accentuate making own choices), this exercise may be insightful for advanced students and practitioners. Research does not have to be anything special we do on top of our busy lives, and in fact we all research. Each of us researches through reflecting on our work with clients, so I suggest exploring in a dialogic way with our therapists, colleagues, and friends what we have researched in the last six months. What topics were we excited about, felt compelled to do some reading on, or sign up to a workshop on? Could we enhance our understanding of these topics by bringing our own experiences and writing about them? This method suggests that we look back at things we are already researching to bring insights that go beyond what we know.

The research question is an unfinished gestalt. It is our choice whether we want to grapple with it for the next few months or years. I was confident when starting my PhD programme that I would write something like a memoir of my already lived experiences. This was a very naive wish as each of the chapters brought me into the field where not only most of my unfinished gestalts resurfaced, but also I was surrounded by my own shame and vulnerability to a greater extent than I ever anticipated. The choice of the struggle needs consideration of the support and time a researcher has for living, breathing, and dreaming their research question.

The type of question, its interest, and focus will determine what methodology should be applied.

7.2.2 Choosing a methodology for a research study

Although this book promotes autoethnographic approaches to research, many research questions in gestalt therapy will not point to this methodology. For auto-ethnographic methodology, a research study must include a critical analysis of the culture and be focused on personal experiences.

Autoethnography is a study of culture, so we should use it if we want to critically explore the field. Similarly to gestalt therapy, it starts with the exploration of individual experiences as co-emerging within particular field conditions and leads to the deconstruction of the field. This does not need to be the only focus of a study, but the analysis of autoethnographic studies will include reflections on the background that energised the emergent figure.

When it comes to the inclusion of personal experiences, it is important that the researchers ask themselves if they naturally like to self-disclose. If you are a therapist who brings your own experiences into a session in an enriching way, then you are probably able to recreate this in your writing. If, however, this level of openness is not comfortable or preferred, I would suggest that you study other approaches that are less revealing. Although it would be hard to convince a gestalt audience that any research study would not be a piece of personal work, there are many approaches that do not require us to focus solely on ourselves, and hence offer a more comfortable approach to disclosure.

Of the many methodological approaches, some are more suitable to gestalt therapy. Each of the teachers of research methodologies offers their own port-folio of methodologies based on the needs of the training group, and their own interest and academic positioning. Amongst the methodologies that I studied and recommend to my students are relational phenomenological approaches (Finlay and Evans, 2009; Finlay, 2011), phenomenological and heuristic approaches (Moustakas, 1990; Sela-Smith, 2002; Todres, 2007), and alchemical hermeneutics (Romanyshyn, 2007). While relational approaches start the exploration from the emerging interaction, the heuristic approach provides a well-described method for studying a phenomenon that we choose to explore. Alchemical hermeneutics focuses on the social unconscious and I usually recommend it in a transpersonal training.

Methodology determines the set of methods we may use (e.g. scientific experi-ment, interviews, or research journal), and in autoethnography researchers are flexible to choose any methods that can produce the best insights and answers to the research question. The following section explains each of the methods I used in the creation of this book.

7.3 Choosing methods – digging around: personal documents, observations, field notes

Whilst ethnographic methods may include descriptions of activities, events, settings, behaviours, conversations (LeCompte and Schensul, 2010), as well as the researcher's feelings and research process notes (Richardson, 2000), autoethnographic research starts with experiences as located within *shifting relationships of power* (Grant, Short and Turner, 2013). Next, I have included a diverse set of methods, which comprise all the elements mentioned earlier. I have artificially divided the generation of data (*experience*) from the analysis of the data (*discourse*).

The creative approach offered by autoethnography gives an invitation, permission, and even a demand to choose a variety of methods that provide a rich description of the studied experiences. The aim is not to seek the truth as there can be no claim that memories are true, false, accurate, or inaccurate (Ellis, 2004). In line with Deleuze and Patton (2004), I believe that each act of remembering creates a new sense of that memory, hence is not a study of the past experiences, but current and situational remembering (me in the past and me in here-and-now).

The diversity of methods I applied to write this book includes field notes (autobiography, research journal, family diagram, pictures, and drawings), and interviews with my mother and sister. Each of them was used to create a view of a situation that I wanted to describe and then narrowed down using the data analysis procedure (see Section 7.5).

My field notes include four types of data: autobiography including the family diagram, research journal, drawings, and photographs. The research journal includes thoughts and feelings related to the research process, including notes from my academic supervisions and meetings with other professionals. The writing of the autobiography of embodiment was a necessary part of my designing the research as a single case study (in an autoethnographic, not a clinical, way). These sources of data are illustrated by photographs and drawings which may help to overcome the difficulty of explaining the human body through words alone. When writing my research, I employed Pillow's (2003) *uncomfortable reflexivity* which encourages researchers to maintain uncertainty in knowing, as a way of capturing the plurality of my voices (Grant and Zeeman, 2012), the ambiguity of competing body sensations, needs, theories, emotions, and thoughts.

7.3.1 Autobiography

When writing the autobiography, I focused on *epiphanies* (Bochner and Ellis, 1992), moments of significant importance and a further description of these moments and their background. My goal was to describe each of these moments from the point of view of the character that is inherently divided inside. Autobiographical work can help to illuminate *hidden voices* (Coffey, 2004): the *voices* inside me, the selves which I have less access to, which are repressed both emotionally and culturally. However, when describing my family's past, I decided to use some fiction to understand the characters better. For example, considering the background to my mother's experiences, I wrote a short story of a nomadic tribe of Vlachs that her family comes from. Vlachs settled in the Beskidy mountains, gave up their nomadic life, and merged with the structure of 18th-century aristocratic Poland. Most of the autobiography is based, however, on my own experiences as I remembered them or reconstructed them in the process of creation. Having made all these steps has not allowed me to escape from the culture that I am informed by or step aside from all of my prejudices; an autobiographical way of writing has many benefits, but at the end of the day it is a single person story and an invitation to dialogue.

"I start with my physical feelings, thoughts, and emotions", writes Ellis (2004, p. XVII) about her embodied autoethnographic processes that seem very similar to gestalt methodology. When writing my autobiography, I selected a number of methods to enhance the autoethnographic angle. With some of them, I started with a body sensation and that led me to understand more about my past and past generations. In line with agential realism (see the preceding chapter), I trusted the intra-action to emerge through embodied contextual experiences. I aimed at contradicting the linear, teleological representation by being guided by my current embodied need and remembered sensations that have become contextualised through the embodied themes from my childhood. The true starting point was an introspecting inhalation, bringing focus and awareness to my *body schema*: "My body becomes a text embodying what I have lived through, witnessed, and experienced" (Metta, 2013, p. 497). For example, Chapter 3 begins from a phenomenological exploration of a sensation, but also includes references to how I embodied current issues. Some autoethnographic paragraphs were written more conceptually, however, providing a meaningful context to the data presented in this study. The connection between phenomenological sensations and sociopolitical data is shown throughout this study. Each piece of sociopolitical data was gathered through a literature review and discussions with research participants, supervisors, and colleagues until a particular sensuous experience was contextualised. This approach can illuminate the subtle and profound relationship between the body and *ethno* that might have been missed if trying to approach narratives of embodiment in interviews only.

7.3.2 Research journal

A research journal is similar to autobiography, the only difference being that the events are recorded on a regular basis soon after taking place (Iida et al., 2012). My research journal contains details of relationally co-constructed body sensations, thoughts, experiences and, most importantly, insights related to my research project. I have been writing my research journal since 2012. It includes: thoughts from attending conference presentations and workshops; notes about research processes in my personal therapy sessions and clinical supervisions; dreams; descriptions of experiences; poems; insights from my clients; and interactions with students attending my bodywork classes. Additional insights are through meetings with other professionals at conferences and in academic and clinical supervisions (see Section 7.4). What I realised in the process of writing was that the journal would be a compilation of notes undertaken during my supervision, after the work with clients, in Evernote, on conference pads, and the journal itself.

7.3.3 Drawings of my embodiment

Writing my research journal and autobiography, I decided to include 11 drawings that illustrate my own body postures with some of the significant people written about in this study. The creation of the drawings, and later the front cover, was a collaborative work with an artist and illustrator, Anna Taterka, that took several revisions to make sure that the drawings adequately show the feelings and embodiments behind each situation, whilst not allowing any other people to be identified or feel caricatured.

Human figure drawings are a popular way of showing embodied human interactions. Spry (2006) argues that embodied methodologies and writings should include more creative forms to enter the liminal space between *somatic and semantic*. I believe that by including drawings of embodiment and the best possible language to describe body sensations and postures, I have built another bridge between paper and *flesh*.

For these reasons, I considered using a video to record discussions. However, I decided not to go ahead with this as I felt a camera would be likely to impact adversely on the intimate nature of my interviews.

7.3.4 Family diagram

Although initially I planned to use the genogram, a family diagram that shows the emotional and transgenerational influences (Butler, 2008), I realised that the genogram methodology and analysis requires special training in systemic therapy that I do not have. Instead, I used a kinship diagram (Chang, 2008, p. 82), which is often used in autoethnography to map a family's connections. The inclusion of the diagram may add some clarity for the reader and quick reference when required. The names for all present generations were anonymised, while my grandparents' generation names are actual. The diagram is shown as Figure 1.1 (Section 1.3).

7.3.5 Family photographs

As part of the interviews at my family home (see Section 7.3.6), I brought some photographs and asked my mother and sister how they perceived the situations captured in them. Furthermore, in close consultation with them, I selected seven of these photographs for inclusion in my thesis as they helped to illustrate the described content. As the camera's view is no longer considered, in ethnography, as objective (Banks, 1998), I collected some of the information about the photographs that helped me to make decisions about inclusion and exclusion, in accordance with the four elements described by Chalfen (1998, p. 217) in Figure 7.1.

Figure 7.1 describes what Barthes (2000) calls *studium* (the contextual analysis of a photograph). However, my autoethnographic focus led me to attend mainly to the subjective quality of the photograph (*punctum*). "Punctum is that accident which pricks me (but also bruises me, is poignant to me)", writes Barthes (Ibidem, p. 27). The *punctum* is the reason that each of the photographs was selected. I described the *punctum* and *studium* of some of the photographs, leaving some of them to play only an illustrative role, for example, Figure 1.2 (Section 1.3) when introducing my mother.

7.3.6 Interviews

Interviews in autoethnographic research can allow new insights into our past. They enable stories to be collected and viewed from different perspectives, and show various ways of remembering the same events. As a relational therapist and a contextual epistemologist, I believe that we live and grow through and in our relationships.

Between summer 2016 and summer 2017, I met first with my mother and then with my sister to ask them questions about my embodiment and gain a greater understanding of my childhood and culture. As my closest living family members,

Planning the event

- Who chose the photographic event? Who brought and owned the camera? What kind of equipment was used and why?

On camera and behind camera

- What is taking place in the photograph and what took place before the camera? Who decided on this particular photo? What was the setting, attitudes, bodily sensations?

Editing events

- Who developed the photograph? Who chose the particular picture being used?

Exhibition events

- How are the photographs being displayed and why? On what occasions are the family albums being shown or revisited? Who owns the album/collection?

Figure 7.1 Describing family photographs

they were present throughout the majority of the experiences described in my autobiography. The interviews took place in my family home in Poland in an undisturbed time that lasted almost two hours with my mother, and one hour with my sister. I met with them ahead of the interview and after the interview to discuss the ethical implications of providing me with the consent to include them in my writing.

Ellis (2004) notices varying degrees of intimacy and participant engagement in conducting autoethnographic research. While *reflexive dyadic* interviews are similar to traditional interviews, with the researcher asking the questions and the participants answering, *co-constructed interviews* enable more mutuality in creating the stories and generating the data between two people. My interviews were somewhere on a continuum between reflexive dyadic and co-constructed (Ellis, 2004), and I reviewed the method during each interview. Although both types of interview seem to be similar in their constructionist philosophy, the practical difference may be significant. For example, with my mother, the interview was mainly based on my questions that unfolded along with the story. It was a very moving and profound moment that significantly changed our relationship. At the end of the interview we both cried, hugged, and said how much we love each other. The interview with my sister was co-constructed with her asking me questions and challenging me a couple of times.

When conducting the interviews, I subscribed to *interembodied listening*: "When the words show me something 'more' that involves a bodily sense of being present to a whole situation" (Todres, 2007, p. 39). This approach enables the researcher to formulate questions, points of interest, and to deepen the intimacy and quality of relationship with the interviewees. Within autoethnography there is no need for an interview script as used in quantitative research (Taylor, 2005, p. 45), and I only had a number of prompt questions in my head in case we got stuck. Hence, the interviews were relatively unstructured, guided (Finlay and Evans, 2009) only by the interviewees and the interviewer's bodily presence and some prompt questions. I believe that by interviewing my closest family members, I generated a more intimate, embodied portrait of myself beyond the possibilities of a single person analysis.

As the interviews were conducted in my mother tongue, Polish, I transcribed and translated the parts I decided to use. I believe that the possible alternative of hiring an interpreter would not fit the intimacy and epistemology of my research study. I decided to use parts of the interviews that illustrated or challenged the theories included in the preceding chapters.

The interview process in this study is shown in Figure 7.2 (for information on how the process looks from the interviewee's perspective, please see Figure 7.3).

Although I included some topics in this book that my mother or sister described as uncomfortable to share, I had several discussions with them about how to present these topics before they granted their full consent. The ongoing consent that I offered was part of my ethical care for my mother and sister, and some of the other people that I described.

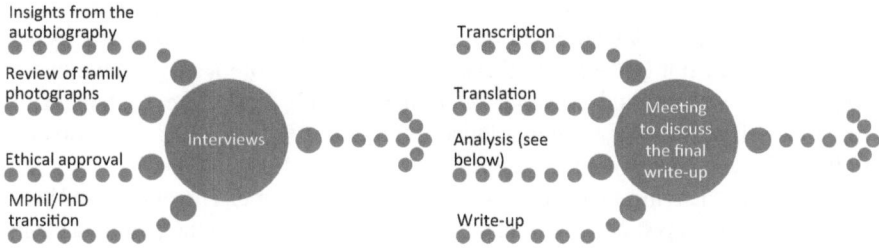

Figure 7.2 The interview process

7.4 Ethical care for participants

Before conducting any research study, or in fact any work with people, we must consider the impact our action will have on them. Autoethnographic research may initially seem not that complicated ethically, as it is the researcher who needs to give the main consent, but there are several issues to consider both relating to the researcher's own safety and wellbeing, and impact on other people indicated in the research study.

Autoethnographic methods seek to enrich the studied phenomenon by including close and intimate descriptions of relationships as well as dialogues (Ellis, 2007; Ellis and Rawicki, 2013). In my research study, I included several groups of participants: myself; my mother, sister, and deceased father; one member of my wider family circle; two clients; five workshop participants; and eight friends and 12 professionals who supported me on my way to becoming a gestalt therapist.

Two participants signed detailed consent forms; six participants were consulted by email; while my friends from childhood and some specialists who worked with my body did not require specific consent due to their episodic role in the research study.

What follows is a description of the participant groups involved in my research and the ethical concerns relating to each. Autoethnographic research studies require special ethical considerations due to their intimate, personal, and relational character. I have therefore applied embodied relational ethics alongside the more standardised requirements of qualitative research studies. Ellis (2007) differentiates between three types of ethics in academic research: procedural, situational, and relational. While the first three sections describe situational and relational ethics mostly applied to the work with participants, procedural ethics is described in the following section. The last section describes situational, embodied ethics and issues that arose when writing various chapters of this research study.

7.4.1 Researcher

Autoethnographic research studies aim at showing the vulnerability of the researcher. Anonymity is not possible unless the researcher decides to use a pseudonym, but this will have an impact on his or her research career and the dialogue with audiences (Etherington, 2005, p. 143). Chapters that emerged in the process of writing include topics that are usually difficult to share: sensitive feelings, family dynamics, or the development of my own sexuality. My clients, students, and colleagues may not be aware of these topics, and therefore it might have had an impact on my work and personal relationships with them. The content of my research will prevent me from making any career in a Polish public institution due to the attitudes towards gender studies (see Section 4.1.4).

There is no denying that this process was uneasy for me. The essence of being an embodied therapist and an autoethnographer is to attend to the pain and shame evoked through this process (Etherington, 2005). However, there are certain steps autoethnographers can take to minimise the emotional impact on themselves and on others. It is the balance of support and critical feedback that can shape a research study and also protect the researcher. During my research study, I presented and discussed my data, not only with my research supervisors, but also with my colleagues, through agreed unpaid support sessions and through paid clinical supervisions. In these meetings, I addressed the possible impact my research may have on myself, my clients, and the participants. All these instances are also bound by a clinical confidentiality agreement and by belonging to a professional therapeutic association.

Life and research are full of ethical challenges on a day-to-day basis, and as a psychotherapist I feel equipped for them. For ethical concerns, I find it insightful to use what Frolic (2011, p. 372) describes as *embodied epistemology* or *mindful epistemology in ethics consultation*. Analysing embodiment on three levels, individual, social, and political, she provides indications of how to enhance ethics through embodiment. I found four particular points useful for my research study:

- paying attention to our embodied gut reactions whilst discussing them with our colleagues and supervisors can minimise our being misled;
- using embodied language in order to make us more aware of relational concerns;
- respect for the embodiment of the people we dialogue with;
- feeling into and addressing any hidden politics and inequalities.

Frolic's (2011) suggestions for using situational ethics places emphasis on embodied sensations and the embodiment of relationships. In an interview with Dick Marivoet, Serge Prengel suggests that the connection to our senses can directly impact ethical decisions: "To the extent that we are connected to our body's senses, our felt senses, then we are much more likely to be ethical" (Marivoet, 2017). By attending to the embodied field, I was able to care for both research participants better as well as for myself. Decisions made in this way enabled me to connect to others through my *flesh*, and to seek the support of my colleagues and supervisors in helping me to become more aware of my *body schema*. This approach helped me to live the *morality* ethics (Grant, 2010), catalysing the integration of my life and research, through embodiment. Etherington (2007) suggests applying reflexivity to ethics, understood in a dialogic way as both awareness of and as a vulnerable sharing of power between researcher and participants. She suggests dialoguing ethical dilemmas with participants, also an invitation to undertake more relational research. These guidelines were particularly useful when I wrote the chapters that included both current situations, such as the break-up of my relationship, and past situations such as transgenerational impact and interviews with my mother and sister.

7.4.2 Mother, sister, and father

Inviting family members to take part in research is problematic, as it requires special ethical consideration. Confidentiality is not possible unless an author decides to stay anonymous (Etherington, 2005, p. 143). I interviewed my mother and sister at our family home in Poland. These interviews were digitally recorded and safely stored, transcribed, and translated by myself (see Section 7.5).

Relational ethics is a reminder that the connections we build during the research process are important and may have a lifelong impact on the participants as well as ourselves (Ellis, 2007); working with one's family, this is a given. In the next section, I describe how I see relational research being consented to, anonymized, and presented. For the interviews, I decided to invite my mother and sister as they are the only remaining close family to me, and they have witnessed me from birth to the present. I initially discussed the concept with them two and a half years before the interviews. They appeared enthusiastic; however, my sister was worried about how emotional this would be. There was no reimbursement offered, nor expected. Figure 7.3 shows the process from the interviewees' perspective.

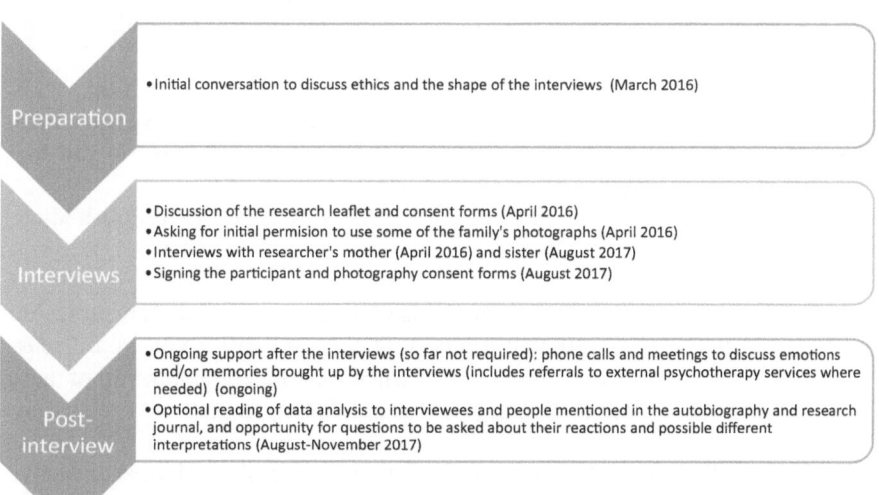

Figure 7.3 Interview process from the interviewee's perspective

I began the interviews by reminding my mother and sister of the research and asking whether they still felt comfortable taking part and being recorded. In line with Miller and Bell (2012) and Etherington (2007), I believed that my family members would not be able to provide informed consent without having direct experience of what they were consenting to. The ongoing process was an invitation to discuss the outcomes of the interviews and acceptable ways in which the data would be presented. I made decisions to exclude some parts of the discussions in my writing. This was guided bodily, for example, on feeling a shrinking sensation in my body. I offered an ongoing type of consent that was renegotiable throughout the research process (Etherington, 2005, 2007; Miller and Bell, 2012). It included a break clause (Finlay and Evans, 2009), allowing my family members to alter information provided, up until our last meeting that we held in November 2017. This meeting was devoted to reading and translating parts of my thesis and I asked for my family's reactions and suggestions on how to present the data. The final video call also included showing family photographs chosen in relation to the text and asking for their feelings and thoughts on them. This opportunity was also used as a space to voice all the different possible interpretations of the data collected (see Section 7.5).

I was prepared for the interviews to bring up both joyful as well as sad memories, but I underestimated the impact of such close conversations with my loved ones. It was the first time I truly listened to my mother, asking her questions about us and her. In my research proposal, I wrote "I will make sure I look after the wellbeing of participants", but this was in a Levinian way, requisitioned by the face of the other (Levinas, 2012, p. 214). Through this meeting, we created the atmosphere of care that seems to last. In fact, we addressed the long-standing distance between the two of us that was difficult to breach in the routines of our life. The following transcription comes from the ending of the interview:

> [AK] **I think it is enough of these questions, mother, but I have one more. How was it meeting me for these almost two hours? How do you feel as we are ending?**
>
> [My mother] I feel as if a stone has fallen down from my heart [Polish idiom for feeling relief].
>
> **Aha.**
>
> You know I want to talk to you. I want to talk to you, but sometimes do not know how, you know? Which topics would entice you to a discussion? I value our discussion and like when we talk. I remember all of these moments when you come closer and share with me as they make me happy.

I think the relief my mother mentioned relates to the quality of intimacy that we created through difficult subjects that we both brought. It opened a new way of communication between us that seems to have a lasting effect.

The interview with my sister started from an apprehensive place that just showed the degree of difficulty and intimacy that we were approaching:

[AK] We will talk about me as a child, about my embodiment. Hmm, I feel tense.

[My sister] Yes, me too.

Hm?

It is hard to decide to move to these times. I can hear my children playing [her two boys are playing in a room next to us], their voices, something so nice and homely and feel as if I was about to return to this land that is frightening.

Oh.

Instantly I feel like crying when I think about this place. Even now the memory is hard to stand.

Oh . . .

You are inviting me to hell [laughter].

You know what? Perhaps we should not go there if it is so difficult for you.

Hmmm, easy . . . I peek there every now and then anyway [laughter].

Ah, okay [laughter].

But it is an impossible place for children to leave. I know this now, looking at my own.

As my sister is also a gestalt psychotherapist, she sees the value in approaching the difficulty of this subject. It is an example of how the ongoing consent is negotiated minute-by-minute in relational ethics. There is no definite procedure that can teach how to behave while doing fieldwork, and so relational ethics helps as it prioritises the relationship and participants' integrity over the outcome of the research. Reminding my sister about the possibility of withdrawing seemed to offer her the safety that she needed to engage with the data.

Sometime before, I facilitated a similar dialogue with an empty chair, imagining my deceased father there and what he would have said about my research thesis and his place in it. I had mixed sensations of exposure and importance. I think my father would have supported a study that emphasises the necessity of opening a dialogue about the collective imprints we all carry.

Although autoethnographic research can cause ethical concerns about the possible coercion of close family members to be involved in research, I believe the risk was minimal concerning my own family. It is a family in which each person expresses his or her opinion and accepts differences as much as similarities. The ongoing consent and sharing of my writing with my family members reduced the risk of coercion. Before obtaining the final consent, I shared with them the paragraphs that include the description of themselves to see how they would feel should this study be published. I applied a similar practice of sending the paragraphs to the people involved when referencing other people included in this research study.

7.4.3 Wider family, bodywork professionals, and clients

Although I did not interview my wider family nor the clients and professionals who supported me on my journey, they were clearly present in the autobiography, research journal, and/or family diagram, and therefore in this book. Each story is a story of relationship (Etherington, 2007). I also took into consideration people who were deceased and their possible wishes, including the opinions of their relatives, and ethics.

Here, as in the interviews mentioned earlier, I anonymised the data (Ellis, 2007) through the use of:

– pseudonyms
– composite characters
– de-composite characters (for example, describing a part of myself as a separate person)
– changing a scene or plot
– metaphors
– choosing not to publish something.

I consulted my research supervisors on anonymisation, paying special attention to contextual power dynamics (Etherington, 2007) and the possible harm these may cause participants. Special care was given to ensure that the ways of anonymising data did not change the nature of embodied sensations. Honesty and transparency above all are required in autoethnographic and any other research studies.

Furthermore, I sent emails to seven people mentioned in this book to discuss the presentation of their encounter and relationship with me in my thesis before completing the writing. I included their descriptions or quotations of the paragraphs that concerned them, along with the wider context of that particular chapter and the whole thesis. Their replies also helped me to analyse and contextualise the data (see Section 7.5).

The participant inclusion criteria were based on their significance to my development as a gestalt therapist, whilst exclusion criteria included mainly ethical concerns, for example: how to make sure that my writing about a past relationship would not negatively affect my ex-partner. I refrained from including in this research people who may be distressed by an honest discussion about our relationship or who preferred not to take part.

Special consideration needed to be given to how to include insights generated during therapy sessions with my clients. My confidentiality agreement does not allow me to include my clients in research; however, many emotions and insights produced during the research process had an impact on my body during their therapy. I consulted my clinical and academic supervisor and decided to refer only to two past clients, and to include five situations that contained descriptions of workshops that I either facilitated or attended. I anonymised and generalised the experiences from my work so much that consent was not necessary.

There were few other situations when I decided against requesting consent. I have not asked *wujek* Janek for consent as I do not think he would understand the point of writing about and deconstructing masculinity. There is little possibility that he will ever hear about this research or read it, and I found it important to include a description of him to illustrate the formation of my masculinity (see Chapter 3). Furthermore, I have not requested a consent from my first therapist. I experienced her work as verging on abuse and I think it is important to write about it. The fact that in the cases of both *wujek* Janek and my first therapist I write about meetings that took place over 20 years ago should provide enough distance for them not to be recognised or associated with this text.

Reimbursement was not offered; however, with some participants such as clinical supervisors and psychotherapists, I have a professional relationship and paid for their services.

Although my research study involved participants, most of the work was based on myself, my experiences, and my own memories. The purpose of the interviews and the inclusion of other participants was not to study them, but to shed more light on my own development of becoming a gestalt therapist.

7.4.4 Procedural ethics, consent procedures, and data storage

Procedural ethics were discussed and agreed in advance of the research study. They are usually written in codes of ethics and, as a psychotherapist, I am obliged to follow the United Kingdom Council for Psychotherapy's Ethical Principles and Code of Professional Conduct (UKCP, 2009). The key procedural documents to my research are: interview consent form, photography consent form, and the research information sheet. My university requested that I undertake a fieldwork abroad risk assessment and get international insurance, as if going to my family home in a Polish village was more dangerous than studying in England.

Having explained how the information was collected and ethically considered, it is timely to outline the strategy for analysing the collected data.

7.5 Making meaning: analysing stories

In autoethnography the boundary between listening to and analysing stories is blurred (Anderson and Glass-Coffin, 2013). In fact, in every encounter with information, research participants and researchers create a new meaning. In this section, I will detail the way I handled data, from its collection to the end of the doctoral thesis writing process.

I let the complete thesis take shape naturally and did not presuppose the order until late. I wanted to allow plurality and an uncertainty of forms (Grant and Zeeman, 2012). At the same time, I needed to have a methodology for ordering the amount of data this research study produced, and putting the thesis together in a possibly open and flexible way. Working towards it, I differentiated four interlinked stages in this process:

Stage one featured autoethnography as a way of collecting and already interpreting sensuous enculturated experiences. It was a diverse process with each of the chapters starting from a different place, some from creative fictional writings about my family's past, another from a place of uncertainty about the way I work, while other chapters marked important transition points and crises in my life.

The second stage of analysis focused on analysing the above, including adding sections of the transcripts from interviews with my mother and sister; field notes and drawings from my meetings with other bodywork professionals; my autobiography with its drawings; my research journal; and my family diagram and family photographs. At this stage, I analysed each chapter separately. In particular, I focused on the embodiment and the use of sensuous descriptions (Stoller, 1997), bringing together phenomenological attention to bodily experiences with cultural critique. I applied Gadamer's hermeneutic method (2012) as it enables the unique dance between personal sensations and wider relational, cultural, and sociological contexts. As shown in Figure 7.4, my embodiment defined and contributed to the context and then was also illuminated by it. For example, exploring the phenomenological sensation of embodying the heteronormativity in Chapter 4 led to more insights about masculinity and the homophobic culture I was critiquing.

"[C]ulture flows through self and vice versa", write Bochner and Ellis (1996), and my way of using the hermeneutic circle in embodied autoethnographic research is an attempt to capture this flow. Referring to the hermeneutic circle in embodied research, Todres (2007) suggests the flow between "closeness" – body and "distance" – language. Therefore, I studied the interplay of my body sensations (as felt when analysing or when writing in the research journal) with words.

At this stage, I was confronting my assumptions and early findings with my research and clinical supervisors, and colleagues, as well as participants of presentations and workshops facilitated by me during this period. At this stage, all data were already sufficiently anonymised (see Section 7.4).

Stage three of data analysis involved synthesising all the anonymised data and chapters together. Based on the concept of assemblages developed by Deleuze and Guattari (1987), the aim was to create diverse, holistic, and truthful texts.

> Method assemblage is the process of enacting or crafting bundles of ramifying relations that condense presence and (therefore also) generate absence

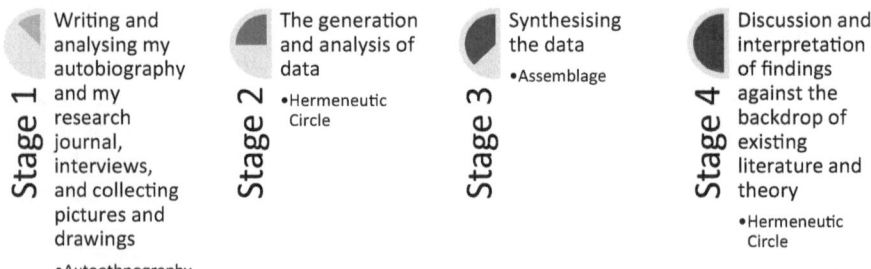

Figure 7.4 Stages of data analysis

by shaping, mediating and separating these. Often it is about manifesting realities out-there and depictions of those realities in-here. It is also about enacting Othernesses.

(Law, 2004, p. 122)

Although I initially considered more traditional and formalised approaches frequently used in qualitative psychology, such as thematic analysis (Braun and Clarke, 2006), assemblages fitted my philosophical interest. In the *multisensory assemblages* (Renold and Mellor, 2013), all voices, including the silent and indeed absent ones, are heard and given space. It was a way of summarising the texts without losing the diversity of the embodied experiences, sensations, and the literature. It is an approach that focused the inseparability of the personal and cultural, whilst accentuating the *differential becoming* between the text, methodology, and the researcher.

In this approach, empirical data sources (interviews, observations, documents, survey data and so forth) are "dredged" to identify the relations and affects that compromise assemblages of bodies, things and social formations within a specific event, and also to assess the capacities that emerge from this assemblage.

(Fox and Alldred, 2017, p. 172)

At this stage, the structure for this research study was agreed to include the assemblage of diversity, the inability to capture sensuous/personal experiences,

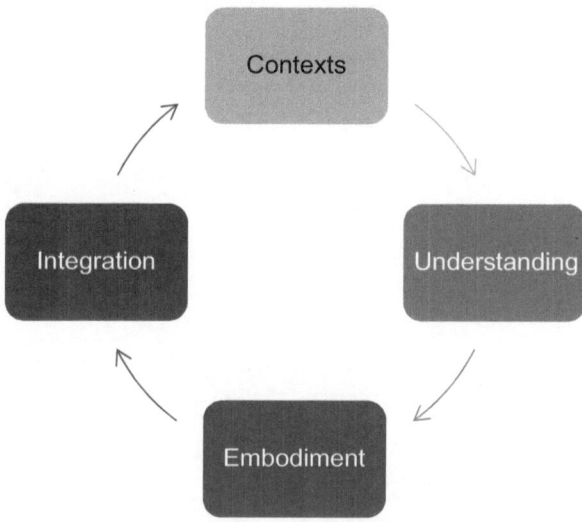

Figure 7.5 A modified version of the Hermeneutic Circle
Source: Bontekoe (1996).

and the development of the argument about the use of collective experiences and prejudices in gestalt therapy training and counselling fully.

Stage four of the analysis started from looking at the text in its totality. Rereading the text in this context and receiving more critique from my colleagues and supervisors, new themes appeared or became more figural. This led to further theorisation and interpretation of my findings against the backdrop of existing literature and theory. The outcome of this stage of analysis was interwoven into the body of the thesis introduction and conclusion, using the hermeneutic circle (see Figure 7.5) as a way of bridging text, experience, theory, and body.

As with any modern car, the engine and electrics of it are complicated. I hope that the last two chapters were not only for qualified mechanics, but also may have encouraged some people to consider being mechanics themselves.

Chapter 8

Conclusion

I wonder if readers of this book, similarly to myself, too often consider the body in psychotherapy from the early childhood developmental perspective, rather than from the wider cultural, relational, and political fields. Even though this tendency is so common, gestalt therapy theory does not limit us to one domain, but considers awareness to be an ongoing process of multiple figure and ground configurations. This is the essence of field theory.

In this book, I advocate for the body as necessarily political and cultural. The invitation to use collective gestalts in gestalt therapy highlights the connection between the body and culture. Each relationship and situation is co-created through a complex web of influences. The awareness of our history and tradition (Gadamer, 2012), collective experiences, and trauma (for example, colonisation) is a gateway, but not a deflection from embodied contact and connection. On the contrary, denial of the history is a source of relational confusion that does not allow us to examine sufficiently our prejudices (Gadamer, 2012), and may lead to deep and lasting psychological traumas such as my father's alcohol abuse. At the same time, history and tradition are alive, powerful and contingent on the here-and-now situation that includes relationships. "What we call history is nothing but the story of the same emotions, the same joys, reproduced across bodies and time", writes Louis (2019, p. 22), but in psychotherapeutic settings there is a hope and an expectation that this history will be rewritten. Both clients and therapists expect it to be a repetition with a difference (Deleuze and Patton, 2004), and psychotherapists need to have the tools and awareness to create such difference. This difference requires the therapists to be wholeheartedly in this process, open and able to rewrite their own history too.

When I began writing this book, I was naive to believe that I would describe experiences from my past, but every chapter opened new experiences and made me attend to my present embodiment of becoming a gestalt therapist. In line with *agential realism* (Barad, 2007), I studied myself as an inter-actively changing object of material-discursive practices that I aimed to describe in this book. The new materialism theory (*agential realism*) that underpins this book gave me the legitimacy and language to reaccentuate the role of *collective experiences* in gestalt therapy. From this perspective, I began my analysis of my psychotherapeutic practice, looking at group work, training, and work with individuals through the lens of my experiences. But are experiences personal? To what degree are my experiences described in this book unique to myself, and where do they illuminate wider social and cultural dynamics? It is not possible to separate the personal and political, therefore each psychotherapeutic encounter should be holistic. For the same reason collective gestalts are so difficult to explore.

With so many benefits, one may ask, why is there so much avoidance of attending to the collective gestalts? The awareness of collective gestalts comes through dialogue that requires us to start with our prejudices (Gadamer, 2012). It is a difficult process of admitting the limitations of our perspective and taking responsibility for how we keep on repeating the collective traumas in current circumstances (*repetition with minimal difference*). That brings another vast difficulty related to the rebalancing of power and more equal distribution of resources, be they the capital in politics or the amount of time each group member takes in group psychotherapy. Finally, the reconfiguration of someone's identity is a difficult process that brings fears and insecurities, and hence there is an investment to avoid it when one can, and several authors have elaborated on how to work with this avoidance. Mindell (1995) calls that fragile place of attending to the difficulty "sitting in the fire", and de Maré, Piper and Thompson (1991) suggest that before dialogue and community are allowed, we need to be able to build conditions necessary for the expression of *hate*. Safety is not a prerequisite for dialogue (de Maré, Piper and Thompson, 1991), but the dialogue itself (Gadamer, 2012). The dialogue, which does not have to be verbal, begins with listening and acknowledgement offered to each side of the conflict: the victim, the perpetrator, and the bystander (Benjamin, 2018). The lasting changes are not created by revolutions that switch the position of power, even though that may be the necessary step. As Polster (1995) suggests, internal freedom is created when each of our parts has a voice; similarly, external peace will begin when we enable ourselves to hear each side of the conflict: Armenian, Azerbaijani, and Georgian; Polish, German, and Jewish; people who oppose and support immigration, women, men, and non-binary female, male, and gender-queer; people from all spectrums of sexual identities (this list is limited to the themes explored in this book).

8.1 Suggestions for theory and practice

8.1.1 Gestalt therapy theory, practice, and training

Considering that phenomenology, for Merleau-Ponty, was the study of the life-world, it is a surprise that in contemporary gestalt therapy, phenomenology is a way of attending to here-and-now sensations that are often reduced to co-emergent, relational, early developmental themes. Although it is in line with *inter-agential co-constitution* (Barad, 2007) to look at a two-person dynamic and early childhood influences, it is also reductionist to restrict the material-discursive context that each phenomenological sensation contains:

The popularisation of psychoanalyzing discourse has sometimes contributed to reducing social issues to psychological ones: [for example] class struggles or the demands of trade unions are chalked up to resolved problems with authority or with the father figure [. . .]. I consider this reduction of the social to the psychological to be a sign of arrogance, as if we were sure to hold the keys to understanding of the world.

(Robine, 2015, p. 220)

A new wave of gestalt therapists addresses this reduction; for example in *New Gestalt Voices*, Bednarek (2017) asks the question of whether her gestalt therapist voted for Brexit. Although there are some therapists who would address political issues, many of us will leave our clients perplexed when we reduce the emerging here-and-now experience to early developmental dynamics. We seem to forget how much prejudice we carry, and that we guide (sometimes out-of-awareness) our clients to interpretations of embodied sensations that make us feel comfortable. I think there are several reasons why gestalt therapy lacks sufficient discussion and training on material-discursive aspects of phenomenology, which include commercialisation of gestalt therapy and the minimally explored legacy of hegemonic masculinity.

Gestalt therapy was not founded just as a method for individual counselling, but as a movement that aimed at social change. Paul Goodman, one of the authors of the founding text in gestalt therapy (Perls, Hefferline and Goodman, 2003), was a well-known social activist, anarchist, and critic of capitalism and modern society (Goodman, 2010). It is the very same capitalism that gave shape to gestalt therapy (Melnick, 2017), exploiting it into the only profitable business that gestalt therapy could easily become: psychotherapy and training; and in that way, it was later reproduced. That marked the move from social and collective issues presented amongst the founders, and reduced the applicability of gestalt therapy to the mother and infant relationship, attachment theories, and relationality that is mainly presented as dyadic, except for sexual transference, which can be made into a triadic Oedipal event (Spagnuolo Lobb, 2009).

Although this book considers only the one-person journey (see Section 8.2), it illustrates how collective gestalts can be brought to the awareness of and worked with in one-to-one, group, and large group therapy. It shows how psychotherapy is necessarily political but also personal, and how many therapeutic encounters are influenced by our sense of social belonging, history, social, and economic circumstances.

In the well-known phrase, "lose your mind come to your senses" (Perls, 2017), lies the definition of gestalt therapy phenomenology that became popular around bioenergetically orientated gestalt therapists (see Chapter 5). Intellectualisations were considered a removal from embodiment, and although one's "truth" was to be found through embodied sensations, they were often interpreted by the facilitators. In the belief that the body will tell its truth through emotions, and that facilitators can create a value- and interpretation-free environment, gestalt therapy was doomed to heteronormativity, racism, middle-class attitudes, or concepts of culture and gender that were left unexplored:

> Emotions are bound up with securing of social hierarchy: emotions become attributes of bodies as a way of transforming what is "lower" or "higher" into bodily traits.
>
> (Ahmed, 2004, p. 4)

Although I am not arguing that all gestalt trainings were highly prejudiced, the structure did not support dismantling the prejudices beyond the awareness and morality of the facilitator, while actively attacking other forms of dealing with collective gestalts and the social hierarchy recreated through them. This structure of shaming trainees for thinking critically was a way to control gestalt communities by charismatic leaders (Philippson, 2014b) that is just another legacy of the unexplored hegemonic masculinity in gestalt therapy.

Hegemonic masculinity is also obsessed with achievement and potency (see Section 3.3.2), hence the choice of early developmental themes that can be easily applied using the bioenergetic model (see Chapter 5). The contrast between the hopelessness, fear, and possibility of failure attending to collective gestalts and the spectacular emotional discharges, tears, and gratitude present in the bioenergetically infused gestalt therapy is large. The work with collective gestalts requires the openness to failure and uncertainty (Staemmler, 1997) that hegemonic masculinity of whatever gender is unable to afford.

Am I then simply suggesting that gestalt therapists abandon the use of phenomenology and focus on the intellectual understanding of field theory? Not at all.

> Merleau-Ponty's sentences convey an implicit sense of belonging to the world, while Foucault's often identify or mobilize elements of resistance and disaffection circulating within modern modalities of experience. The initial connection between these two thinkers across their differences is that both see how perception requires a prior disciplining of the senses in which a rich history of inter-involvement sets the stage for experience.
>
> (Connolly, 2010, p. 187)

Gestalt therapists need to rethink the way they understand and apply phenomenology. As *epoché* in psychotherapy is a discipline that allows us to tune into subtle embodied here-and-now sensations (Spinelli, 2005), we need to have another way of tuning into our collective, prejudiced bodies. Since our culture shapes our bodies and our bodies shape our co-emergent experiences when working with clients, the training of psychotherapists needs to put emphasis on creating conditions that challenge our embodiments of culture and ethics. "Bodies [. . .] acquire orientation through the repetitions of some actions over others" (Ahmed, 2010, p. 247). Emphasis needs to be put on the collective gestalts interwoven both in the culture of the trainings that we offer and in the psychotherapeutic sessions. Instead of feeling comfortable mainly with early developmental interpretations of our clients' embodied sensations, we need to support them to feel their enculturated bodies, recognising that each act of bodily perception contains the inevitable co-emergent mix of embodied sensations and prejudices that we carry.

This is not to be done in a self-punishing way. As shown in various chapters of this book, I have a tendency to blame myself, and other therapists may have it too. Self-punishment and self-attack are the reinforcement of the taboo that lies in addressing collective gestalts in our culture, but they are also representational of anger about social inequality. On the contrary, we need to find support to let ourselves be vulnerable and *deliberately expose* ourselves to *power* (Butler, 2016), where social inequalities are felt bodily, and hence are no longer a taboo, and where emphasis is put on how current structures represent these inequalities (Bordo, 1989). Blame, attack, and anger are, as in any collective gestalt, just a part of it. They are necessary and need to be included; the phenomenology of anger can mark the beginning of a dialogue (de Maré, Piper and Thompson, 1991), but it is *vulnerability* that is the starting point for political and personal changes. The experience of vulnerability allows us to sense the embodied resonance (Frank, 2001) or, using Benjamin's vocabulary, to attend to the *embodied identification* and *empathy* (2018) towards victim, perpetrators, and bystanders. In line with *agential materialism* (Barad, 2007), it is hard to distinguish what comes first: whether it's desire, or vulnerability, or dialogue, or empathy. It is also impossible to create a prescription for how to expand these areas. However, what is clear to me is that psychotherapy, including gestalt therapy, has great potential to combine the attention to sensations, desires, vulnerability, dialogue, and empathy that needs to be understood beyond dyadic and only human-to-human relationships. This will create the change and allow the collective gestalts to be rebalanced.

To summarise, gestalt therapists need to engage in embodied, empathic, and vulnerable dialogues that address the practices that recreate the inequalities in current field conditions. As shown in Chapter 4, the detachment that embodied prejudices offer can be sufficient reason to engage in a dialogue on collective gestalts, and this process took me a few years. Taking the risk of generalising from my own example, there is an interest in the dominant groups to redress social inequalities. The phenomenological sensation of lack and emptiness can be a good enough reason to reach out into the unknown and to fill this gap, but the current consumeristic culture finds competing conceptions on how to fill in that emptiness. The current detached culture that removes us from each other and our communities correlates with the avoidance of collective gestalts and other difficulties that dialogue can present. The inclusion of large groups in the training of psychotherapists should be only one of the places where such dialogue happens.

8.1.2 Case for large groups in teaching counselling and psychotherapy

Although gestalt large groups, to my knowledge, are offered only in one place in the world, they have great potential to help students of counselling and psychotherapy to become aware of the complexity of their diversity and to reduce their fear of attending to their own prejudices.

Social identity theory claims that:

> [R]ole identity change is more likely to occur in organizations or groups that significantly change in size compared to organizations or groups that are relatively stable in size. [. . .] [I]dentity change is a function of changing connectedness of identities within the social structure.
>
> (Stets, 2006, p. 105)

The process of identity change may also correlate with an increased awareness of multiple identities (Stets, 2006), awareness, and ownership of category (salience) as well as increased personal contact (Dovidio, Gaertner and Kawakami, 2003, p. 13), and hence the possibility to change and learn from others. Large groups reorganise social structures of people involved through attention given to collective processes. In large groups, the social meets the personal, and our sense of belonging is called into question.

In particular, large groups could help trainee therapists learn therapeutic skills, to become aware of their diversity, and to build a community in various ways (Kincel, 2015a):

- Therapeutic skills

  - Study group dynamics and processes (Island, 2003)
  - Strengthen students' capacity to tolerate regressive experiences (Pines, 2003). In other words, how to be tuned to others whilst experiencing threats to one's identity (Skynner, 1975, p. 247)
  - Increase capacity to handle separation anxiety (de Maré, Piper and Thompson, 1991)
  - Increase capacity to handle traumatic neuroses (de Maré, Piper and Thompson, 1991)
  - Increase agency and creativity (Skaife and Jones, 2008, p. 208)

- Diversity awareness

  - Expose an ignorant, fixed, and often damaging way of participating in society
  - Develop citizenship (Pines, 2003)
  - [Related to the previous point] Study the large group as a microsociety, experiencing parallel processes (Schneider and Weinberg, 2003, p. 17)
  - Develop links with our socio-cultural environment (de Maré, Piper and Thompson, 1991, p. 10)
  - Create subgrouped support for minorities (Agazarian, 2004; O'Neill, Constantino and Mogle, 2012)
  - Increase competency in handling cultural conflicts (de Maré, Piper and Thompson, 1991, p. 178)

- • Increase complexity of the social identities (Roccas and Brewer, 2002)
- • Change social identity (Burke, 2004)

• Community building (Island, 2003; Pines, 2003).

Some research claims that some large groups (i.e. Large-group awareness training) had no significant effect on participants (Fisher, 1990). Fisher and his team examined Large-Group Awareness Training, looking at the impact on participants' emotional wellbeing and worldview, and found no significant changes. By employing psychometric questionnaires, Fisher and his team were not able to hear individual stories and feel the impact large groups had on participants' lives. Although more recent qualitative studies show the efficiency of large groups (O'Neill, Constantino and Mogle, 2012), more research is needed to elaborate on the full potential and impact of the large group.

In general, large groups assist training therapists to learn new skills, develop awareness of diversity, and build a community. At the same time, gestalt training institutes have not applied this methodology on a larger scale. Similarly in research, large groups have not been studied sufficiently, and the autoethnographic methodology applied in this book offered a unique perspective of discovering collective gestalts through a one-person embodiment.

8.1.3 Interweaving autoethnography and gestalt therapy

Researchers have focused on the importance of evaluating research according to its epistemological stance (Sparkes, 2002a; Willig, 2008). There are various guidelines towards how autoethnographic research should be evaluated, but each of them is based on aesthetic criteria familiar to gestalt therapists. Anderson and Glass-Coffin (2013, pp. 71–79) list five points which constitute the essence of autoethnographic research: visibility of self (its diversity and richness); strong reflexivity; engagement (with oneself and others); vulnerability; and open-endedness/ rejection of finality and closure. A similar list is presented by Richardson (2000), who suggests an evaluation of autoethnography, according to a contribution to understanding, aesthetic merit, reflexivity, emotional or intellectual impact, and lived experience.

I aimed at meeting these features by analysing and writing about data that emerged from my current concerns about my practice but were linked with my past, as a gestalt therapist in the process of becoming. I aimed to make myself visible using a multitude of creative forms, such as dialogues, drawings, photographs, and self-narratives. Bringing the phenomenological method, I started and ended with my embodiment and used it as an aesthetic and ethical tool. "Bodies are more than the stories we tell of them and, therefore, our bodies have the potential to serve as a kind of personal 'check' or 'test' of the stories we tell about them," writes Carless (2010, p. 340). The reflexivity is evidenced through shifting levels of analyses throughout the text. Although they may feel on occasion abrupt, as the timeline and cultural context may change rapidly, my aim was to show the diversity and complexity of reflexivity in any *intra-active constitution*. Reflexivity was deepened when I presented the outcomes of all the findings chapters to other bodies (colleagues, supervisors, research participants). These dialogues were necessary for me to elaborate on my prejudices (Gadamer, 2012) and allowed me to explore my body discursively (Barad, 2007; Butler, 1993). This enhanced the reflexivity and visibility of my selves through the richness of interpretations and perspectives.

The aim of this work was not to show how much I changed and how I moved from being prejudiced to being non-prejudiced, but to illustrate how prejudices are inevitably embedded in our work and private lives, and how we need to find ways of attending to them on a day-to-day basis. How do we notice our prejudices, find support to deal with the shame that these realisations bring, and the self-compassion that we need to move on from them? The analysis of conditions that produce inequalities (Bordo, 1989) is an aim that should be incorporated into each therapy session or relationship, and indeed it is a never-ending process.

The main message in this book, advocating for therapists to discover their collective positioning and to disclose it in the therapeutic relationships as an invitation to shift emerging power dynamics, is similar to the aims that autoethnography has in general (Allen-Collinson, 2013). Is it possible that the methodology had a significant impact on the findings, and what would be the outcomes if another methodology was applied? The methodology had an impact on this research study and the outcomes would be different if another person or even myself tried to replicate the process of this study. Both autoethnography and new materialism are aware of the temporality of each discovery and do not claim to produce generalisable outcomes. The question of the value of this book is therefore left to you. Has it produced enough dialogue between the reader and the text in their *differential becoming*? Would some of the insights impact the way gestalt therapy is practised and theorised? Do you feel enticed to write your own autoethnography?

Even if this book aims at reducing my own prejudices, it is also an evidence of the current restriction of my social positioning. The next section explores some of the limitations.

8.2 What I know I've missed

The research focus on my embodiment carved a perspective that opened some avenues for exploration while closing other possibilities. As methodological alternatives and limitations have been discussed (see Section 7.2.2), here I focus on limitations that relate to the content of this thesis and, more specifically, the issues of race, eco-psychology, and wider engagement with the research participants.

Although through my body I stayed consistent with the theme of collective gestalts, this journey took me towards a wide territory that required an extensive literature review. The exploration was more horizontal than vertical, and as with every map that covers vast areas of land, this research study misses the specifics of some of the discourses that I referred to. My aim and energy were in the con-nection and synthesis of various philosophies, psychotherapeutic, and research methodologies, rather than in-depth critique and analysis.

The strong theme of diversity and equality in gestalt therapy includes reflec-tions, autoethnographic data, and theories on culture, masculinity, and sexuality. What is clearly missed here is the often-silenced collective gestalt of race and its relationship with colonialism and slavery. Although I have a number of rational reasons why race does not feature in this research study, it is my duty to wonder how I have embodied collective racism manifested in the discard of Black, Asian, and minority ethnic people. This includes the limited engagement of psychothera-pists and psychotherapeutic training centres (Jacobs, 2014) with non-white com-munities in the US and England.

Another limitation that also reinforces a stereotype is the lack of dialogue with others and limited dialoguing opportunity with my mother and sister. It is another white men's written perspective that could have been very different should other research participants have been allowed to comment more. I think if I designed this study today, I would be less ambitious about the widespread content and more focused on the relational co-created dynamics of the study's phenomena. Although each chapter was discussed not only during research supervisions but also during lectures, presentations, peer support groups, and other forms of dia-logue that offered challenges, including more people in a dialogical way, ie rela-tional autoethnography or choosing a research methodology that encourages more dialogue and verification, could have benefited this book.

Although I was truthful to the material-discursive phenomenology, I have not engaged much with ecological matters in my writing. Eco-psychology, which accentuates the connection between psychological health and ecology (Rust and Totton, 2012), is missed in this book and would be relevant to sharpen the connec-tions between the new materialism and collective gestalts. This subject could have ignited difficult discussions about how as gestalt therapists we ignore environ-mental concerns and travel thousands of air miles to enable direct contact during our conferences and workshops.

8.3 Ending

This marks an end to over seven years of my professional life. Looking back at it I am reminded of the moment when I came to my research supervisors to request a year break in my doctoral training due to personal difficulties. My supervisors listened to me attentively as I cried and shared my situation, then one of them suggested I take two months when I only write about my pain to see if this could be transferred into an autoethnographic piece. Of course, this writing quickly transformed into a story on collective gestalts and was integrated in some of the chapters of this book.

Autoethnography hurts. As with the advice of my supervisors, it starts from an invitation to write where it hurts, but the process of writing is also painful.

Each birth requires pain. It is also a process that hurts afterwards with the possibility of feeling exposed. Tamas reports on how she feels when her book is praised:

> I feel a brief flash of hope before my throat tightens with the worry that I've over-shared, fooled them, and created expectations that I can't possibly fulfill. This, my therapist explains, is how people with low self-esteem respond to compliments.
>
> (2013, p. 195)

This book is an invitation to explore this pain – starting with the shame of exposure that each of us feels when discovering our own prejudices and ending with autobiographical writing. I hope to offer both an encouragement to engage with the shame and hurt of discovering collective gestalts, but also techniques on how to do it in a way that is safe, practical, and useful. Creating a safe environment where we can experiment with getting to know ourselves through our prejudices is an important task not only for large groups, but also intimate relationships.

The focus on collective gestalts is what I hope people who engage with this book will retain. Gestalt therapy needs to reinstate itself as a valid method to attend to collective issues in training, individual, and group psychotherapy. We need to be able to build bridges that enable communication between people who do not share the same political views and perspectives. Gestalt psychotherapy, with its focus on embodiment, always depending on current field conditions, has a methodology that can enable this. With greater awareness paid to collective gestalts, their dialogical dynamism and the need for empathy and vulnerability to attend to political issues in the consulting room and outside, gestalt therapists have much to offer to facilitate difficult political dialogues. These skills are particularly important in the times of huge political divisions that we live in.

References

Agazarian, Y.M. (2004). *Systems-centered Therapy for Groups*. London: Karnac Books.

Ahmed, S. (2004). *The Cultural Politics of Emotion*. Edinburgh: Edinburgh University Press.

Ahmed, S. (2010). Orientation Matter. In: Coole, D. and Frost, S. (Eds.), *New Materialisms: Ontology, Agency, and Politics*. Durham, NC: Duke University Press, pp. 234–257.

Alexander, J.C. (2004). *Cultural Trauma and Collective Identity*. Berkeley: University of California Press.

Allen-Collinson, J. (2011). Intention and Epoché in Tension: Autophenomenography, Bracketing and a Novel Approach to Researching Sporting Embodiment. *Qualitative Research in Sport, Exercise and Health*, 3, 1: 48–62.

Allen-Collinson, J. (2013). Autoethnography as the Engagement of Self/Other, Self/Culture, Self/Politics, and Selves/Futures. In: Holman Jones, S.L., Adams, T.E. and Ellis, C. (Eds.), *Handbook of Autoethnography*. Walnut Creek, CA: Left Coast Press, Incorporated, pp. 281–299.

Ambroziak, A. (2017). *Premier Szydło z nagrodą „Prawda-Krzyż-Wyzwolenie" wraz z organizacją, która „leczy" z homoseksualności* [Accessed: March 20, 2017].

Amendt-Lyon, N. (2008). Gender Differences in Gestalt Therapy. *Gestalt Review*, 12, 2: 106–121.

Amendt-Lyon, N. (2013). Relational Sexual Issues: Love and Lust in Context. In: Francesetti, G., Gecele, M. and Roubal, J. (Eds.), *Gestalt Therapy in Clinical Practice: From Psychopathology to the Aesthetics of Contact*. Siracusa: Instituto di Gestalt HCC Italy, pp. 583–598.

Amendt-Lyon, N. (2016). *Timeless Experience: Laura Perls's Unpublished Notebooks and Literary Texts 1946–1985*. Newcastle upon Tyne: Cambridge Scholars Publishing.

Anderson, E. (2009). *Inclusive Masculinity: The Changing Nature of Masculinities*. New York: Taylor & Francis.

Anderson, L. and Glass-Coffin, B. (2013). I Learn by Going: Autoethnographic Modes of Inquiry. In: Holman Jones, S.L., Adams, T.E. and Ellis, C. (Eds.), *Handbook of Autoethnography*. Walnut Creek, CA: Left Coast Press, Incorporated, pp. 57–84.

Anzieu, D. (1984). *The Group and the Unconscious*. London: Routledge & Kegan Paul.

Atkinson, P. (1990). *The Ethnographic Imagination: Textual Constructions of Reality*. London: Routledge.

Banks, M. (1998). Visual Anthropology: Image, Object and Interpretation. In: Prosser, J. (Ed.), *Image-based Research: A Sourcebook for Qualitative Researchers*. Philadelphia: Falmer Press, Taylor & Francis Group, pp. 9–23.

Barad, K. (2003). Posthumanist Performativity: Toward an Understanding of How Matter Comes to Matter. *Signs*, 28, 3: 801–831.

Barad, K. (2007). *Meeting the Universe Halfway: Quantum Physics and the Entanglement of Matter and Meaning*. Durham, NC: Duke University Press.

Barad, K. (2011). Nature's Queer Performativity. *Qui Parle: Critical Humanities and Social Sciences*, 19, 2: 121–158.

Barad, K., Dolphijn, R. and van der Tuin, I. (2012). Matter Feels, Converses, Suffers, Desires, Yearns and Remembers. In: Dolphijn, R. and van der Tuin, I. (Eds.), *New Materialism: Interviews & Cartographies*. Ann Arbor: Open Humanities Press, pp. 1–15.

Barber, P. (2006). *Becoming a Practitioner Researcher: A Gestalt Approach to Holistic Inquiry*. London: Middlesex University Press.

Barthes, R. (2000). *Camera Lucida: Reflections on Photography*. London: Vintage Books.

Bartleet, B. (2013). Artful and Embodied Methods, Modes of Inquiry, and Forms of Representation. In: Holman Jones, S.L., Adams, T.E. and Ellis, C. (Eds.), *Handbook of Autoethnography*. Walnut Creek, CA: Left Coast Press, Incorporated, pp. 443–464.

Bartlett, A., King, M. and Phillips, P. (2001). Straight Talking: An Investigation of the Attitudes and Practice of Psychoanalysts and Psychotherapists in Relation to Gays and Lesbians. *The British Journal of Psychiatry*, 179, 6: 545–549.

Bar-Yoseph Levine, T. (2012). *Gestalt Therapy: Advances in Theory and Practice*. Hove: Routledge.

BBC News. (2018). *Poland U-Turn on Holocaust Law*. Available at: www.bbc.co.uk/news/world-europe-44627129. [Accessed: March 20, 2017].

Bednarek, S. (2017). Brexit and Psychotherapy. *New Gestalt Voices*, 28 November [Blog]. Available at: https://newgestaltvoices.org/brexit-and-psychotherapy/ [Accessed: December 1, 2017].

Bednarek, S. (2018). How Wide is the Field? Gestalt Therapy, Capitalism and the Natural World. *British Gestalt Journal*, 27, 2: 8–17.

Beisser, A. (1970). The Paradoxical Theory of Change. In: Fagan, J. and Shepard, I.L. (Eds.), *Gestalt Therapy Now*. New York: Science and Behavior Books, pp. 77–80.

Benjamin, J. (1996). In Defense of Gender Ambiguity. *Gender and Psychoanalysis*, 1, 1: 27–43.

Benjamin, J. (2018). *Beyond Doer and Done To: Recognition Theory, Intersubjectivity and the Third* (Inspection Copy). Oxon and New York: Routledge.

Bennett, J.L. (2010). 'Inocencia': Case Study of a Transgender Woman without Gender Dysphoria Preparing for Gender Reassignment Surgery. *British Gestalt Journal*, 19, 2: 16–27.

Bion, W.R. (1984). *Second Thoughts: Selected Papers on Psychoanalysis*. London: Karnac Books.

Bly, R. (2013). *Iron John*. London: Random House.

Bochner, A.P. and Ellis, C. (1992). Personal Narrative as a Social Approach to Interpersonal Communication. *Communication Theory*, 2, 2: 165–172.

Bochner, A.P. and Ellis, C. (1996). Introduction: Talking over Ethnography. In: Ellis, C. and Bochner, A.P. (Eds.), *Composing Ethnography: Alternative Forms of Qualitative Writing*. Walnut Creek, CA: AltaMira Press, pp. 13–48.

Bocian, B. (2010). *Fritz Perls in Berlin 1893–1933: Expressionism – Psychoanalysis – Judaism*. Wuppertal: EHP.

Bonilla-Silva, E. (2006). *Racism without Racists: Color-Blind Racism and the Persistence of Racial Inequality in the United States*. Lanham, MD: Rowman & Littlefield Publishers.

Bontekoe, R. (1996). *Dimensions of the Hermeneutic Circle*. Atlantic Highlands, NJ: Humanities Press.

Bordo, S. (1989). The Body and the Reproduction of Femininity: A Feminist Appropriation of Foucault. In: Jaggar, A.M. and Bordo, S. (Eds.), *Gender/Body/Knowledge: Feminist Reconstructions of Being and Knowing*. New Brunswick: Rutgers University Press, pp. 13–33.

Bordo, S. (2000). *The Male Body: A New Look at Men in Public and in Private*. New York: Farrar, Straus and Giroux.

Bourdieu, P. (1990a). *In Other Words: Essays Towards a Reflexive Sociology*. Stanford: Stanford University Press.

Bourdieu, P. (2001). *Masculine Domination*. Stanford: Stanford University Press.

Bowlby, J. (1997). *Attachment, Attachment and Loss*. London: Pimlico.

Braidotti, R. (2011). *Nomadic Subjects: Embodiment and Sexual Difference in Contemporary Feminist Theory*. New York: Columbia University Press.

Braidotti, R. (2013). *The Posthuman*. Cambridge: Polity Press.

Braun, V. and Clarke, V. (2006). Using Thematic Analysis in Psychology. *Qualitative Research in Psychology*, 3, 2: 77–101.

Brennan, K.A. and Shaver, P.R. (1995). Dimensions of Adult Attachment, Affect Regulation, and Romantic Relationship Functioning. *Personality and Social Psychology Bulletin*, 21, 3: 267–283.

Brothers, D. (2007). *Toward a Psychology of Uncertainty: Trauma-centered Psychoanalysis*. New York: Taylor & Francis.

Brothers, D. (2017). If Freud Were a Woman: Gender, Uncertainty, and the Psychology of Being Human. *Psychoanalytic Inquiry*, 37: 419–424.

Brownell, P. (2014). C'mon Now, Let's Get Serious about Research. *Gestalt Review*, 18, 1: 6–22.

Buber, M. (2004). *I and Thou*. London: Continuum.

Bunker, B.B. and Alban, B.T. (1997). *Large Group Interventions: Engaging the Whole System for Rapid Change*. San Francisco: Jossey-Bass.

Bunker, B.B. and Alban, B.T. (2006). *The Handbook of Large Group Methods: Creating Systemic Change in Organizations and Communities*. San Francisco: Jossey-Bass.

Burke, P.J. 2004. Identities and Social Structure: The 2003 Cooley-Mead Award Address. *Social Psychology Quarterly*, 67, 1: 5–15.

Butler, J. (1993). *Bodies that Matter: On the Discursive Limits of 'Sex'*. New York: Routledge.

Butler, J. (2011). *Gender Trouble: Feminism and the Subversion of Identity*. New York: Routledge.

Butler, J. (2016). Rethinking Vulnerability and Resistance. In: Butler, J., Gambetti, Z. and Sabsay, L. (Eds.), *Vulnerability in Resistance*. Durham, NC: Duke University Press, pp. 12–27.

Butler, J.F. (2008). The Family Diagram and Genogram: Comparisons and Contrasts. *American Journal of Family Therapy*, 36, 3: 169–180.

Carless, D. (2010). Who the Hell was That? Stories, Bodies and Actions in the World. *Qualitative Research in Psychology*, 7, 4: 332–344.

Carman, T. (1999). The Body in Husserl and Merleau-Ponty. *Philosophical Topics*, 27, 2: 205–226.

Carman, T. (2008). *Merleau-Ponty*. London: Routledge.

Chalfen, R. (1998). Interpreting Family Photographs as Pictorial Communication. In: Prosser, J. (Ed.), *Image-based Research: A Sourcebook for Qualitative Researchers*. Philadelphia: Falmer Press, Taylor & Francis Group, pp. 214–234.

Chang, H. (2008). *Autoethnography as Method*. Walnut Creek, CA: Left Coast Press.

Clarke, V., Ellis, S., Peel, E. and Riggs, D.W. (2010). *Lesbian, Gay, Bisexual, Trans and Queer Psychology: An Introduction*. Cambridge: Cambridge University Press.

Clemmens, M. (2010). *Workshop: Gestalt Therapy as Embodied Relational Practice*. Edinburgh: Edinburgh Gestalt Institute.

Clemmens, M. (2012). The Interactive Field – Gestalt Therapy as Embodied Relational Dialogue. In: Bar-Yoseph Levine, T. (Ed.), *Gestalt Therapy: Advances in Theory and Practice*. London: Routledge, pp. 39–48.

Clemmens, M. and Bursztyn, A. (2005). Culture and Body. In: Levine Bar-Yoseph, T. (Ed.), *The Bridge: Dialogues across Cultures*. Metairie, New Orleans, LA: Gestalt Institute Press, pp. 15–21.

CNN. (2006). *Ex-Gay Guru Richard Cohen Demonstrating His Reparative Therapy Techniques on CNN*. Available at: www.youtube.com/watch?v=VtGouVqsmsg [Accessed: November 1, 2017].

Coffey, A. (2004). Autobiography. In: Lewis-Beck, M.S., Bryman, A. and Liao, T.F. (Eds.), *Encyclopedia of Social Science Research Methods*. Thousand Oaks, CA: SAGE Publications, Incorporated, pp. 46–47.

Collins English Dictionary. (2014). *Definition of 'Ethno-'*. Available at: www.collinsdictionary.com/dictionary/english/ethno [Accessed: November 1, 2017].

Collinson, D. and Hearn, J. (1996). 'Men' at 'Work': Multiple Masculinities/Multiple Workplaces. In: Mac an Ghaill, M. (Ed.), *Understanding Masculinities: Social Relations and Cultural Arenas*. Buckingham: Open University Press, pp. 61–76.

Collinson, D.L. (1992). *Managing the Shopfloor: Subjectivity, Masculinity and Workplace Culture, Vol. 36*. Berlin: Walter de Gruyter.

Committee on Nomenclature and Statistics of the American Psychiatric Association. (1968). *DSM-II: Diagnostic and Statistical Manual of Mental Disorders*. Washington, DC: American Psychiatric Association.

Connolly, W.F. (2010). Materialities of Experience. In: Coole, D. and Frost, S. (Eds.), *New Materialisms: Ontology, Agency, and Politics*. Durham, NC: Duke University Press, pp. 178–200.

Coole, D. (2010). The Inertia of Matter and the Generativity of Flesh. In: Coole, D. and Frost, S. (Eds.), *New Materialisms: Ontology, Agency, and Politics*. Durham, NC: Duke University Press, pp. 92–115.

Coole, D. and Frost, S. (2010). Introducing the New Materialism. In: Coole, D. and Frost, S. (Eds.), *New Materialisms: Ontology, Agency and Politics*. Durham, NC: Duke University Press, pp. 1–45.

Cornell, W.F. (2003). The Impassioned Body: Erotic Vitality and Disturbance in Psychotherapy. *British Gestalt Journal*, 12, 2: 97–124.

Corona, G., Petrone, L., Mannucci, E., Mansani, R., Balercia, G., Krausz, C., Giommi, R., Forti, G. and Maggi, M. (2005). Difficulties in Achieving vs Maintaining Erection: Organic, Psychogenic and Relational Determinants. *International Journal of Impotence Research*, 17, 3: 252–258.

Crocker, S.F. (1999). *A Well Lived Life: Essays in Gestalt Therapy*. Santa Cruz: Gestalt Press.

Datta, A. (2009). This is Special Humour: Visual Narratives of Polish Masculinities on London's Building Sites. In: Burrell, K. (Ed.), *Polish Migration to the UK in the 'New' European Union: After 2004*. Abingdon: Taylor & Francis, pp. 189–210.

Davies, D. and Aykroyd, M. (2002). Sexual Orientation and Psychological Contact. In: Wyatt, G. and Sanders, P. (Eds.), *Contact and Perception*. Herefordshire: PCCS Books, pp. 221–233.

de Maré, P. (1975). The Politics of Large Groups. In: Kreeger, L. (Ed.), *The Large Group: Dynamics and Therapy*. London: Karnac Books, pp. 145–158.

de Maré, P., Piper, R. and Thompson, S. (1991). *Koinonia: From Hate through Dialogue to Culture in the Larger Group*. London: Karnac Books.

Deaux, K. and Burke, P. (2010). Bridging Identities. *Social Psychology Quarterly*, 73, 4: 315–320.

Deleuze, G. and Guattari, F. (1987). *A Thousand Plateaus: Capitalism and Schizophrenia*. Minneapolis: University of Minnesota Press.

Deleuze, G. and Patton, P. (2004). *Difference and Repetition*. London: Bloomsbury Academic.

Denzin, N.K. (2013). *Interpretive Autoethnography*. Los Angeles, London, New Delhi, Singapore, Washington, DC: SAGE Publications.

Dickinson, T., Cook, M., Playle, J. and Hallett, C. (2014). Nurses and Subordination: A Historical Study of Mental Nurses' Perceptions on Administering Aversion Therapy for 'Sexual Deviations'. *Nursing*, 21, 4: 283–293.

Dovidio, J.F., Gaertner, S.L. and Kawakami, K. (2003). Intergroup Contact: The Past, Present, and the Future. *Group Processes & Intergroup Relations*, 6, 1: 5–21.

Duffy, N. (2018). European Parliament Condemns Gay 'Cure' Therapy and Tells EU Member States to Ban It. *PinkNews*. Available at: www.pinknews.co.uk/2018/03/01/european-parliament-condemns-gay-cure-therapy-and-tells-eu-member-states-to-ban-it/ [Accessed: November 1, 2019].

Edemariam, A. (2017). *'I Don't Know Who I Am Without It': The Truth about Long-term Antidepressant Use*. Available at: www.theguardian.com/society/2017/may/06/dont-know-who-am-antidepressant-long-term-use [Accessed: November 3, 2017].

Eiden, B. (1998). The Use of Touch in Psychotherapy. *Self & Society*, 26, 2: 3–8.

Eiden, B. (2011). The History of Body Psychotherapy: An Overview. In: Young, C. (Ed.), *The Historical Basis of Body Psychotherapy*. Galashields: Body Psychotherapy Publications, pp. 39–48.

Elise, D. (1998). Gender Repertoire: Body, Mind, and Bisexuality. *Psychoanalytic Dialogues*, 8, 3: 353–371.

Ellis, C. (1995). *Final Negotiations: A Story of Love, Loss, and Chronic Illness*. Philadelphia: Temple University Press.

Ellis, C. (2004). *The Ethnographic I: A Methodological Novel about Autoethnography*. Walnut Creek, CA: AltaMira Press.

Ellis, C. (2007). Telling Secrets, Revealing Lives: Relational Ethics in Research with Intimate Others. *Qualitative Inquiry*, 13, 1: 3–29.

Ellis, C., Adams, T.E. and Bochner, A.P. (2010). Autoethnography: An Overview. *Forum: Qualitative Social Research*, 12, 1: 1–18.

Ellis, C. and Rawicki, J. (2013). Collaborative Witnessing of Survival during the Holocaust: An Exemplar of Relational Autoethnography. *Qualitative Inquiry*, 19, 5: 366–380.

Emery, F.E. and Trist, E.L. (1960). Socio-Technical Systems. In: Churchman, C.W. and Verhuls, M. (Eds.), *Management Sciences, Models and Techniques*. London: Pergamon Press, pp. 83–97.

Essén, A. and Värlander, S.W. (2013). The Mutual Constitution of Sensuous and Discursive Understanding in Scientific Practice: An Autoethnographic Lens on Academic Writing. *Management Learning*, 44, 4: 395–423.

Etherington, K. (2003). *Trauma, the Body and Transformation: A Narrative Inquiry*. London: Jessica Kingsley Publishers.

Etherington, K. (2005). *Becoming a Reflexive Researcher*. London: Jessica Kingsley Publishers.

Etherington, K. (2007). Ethical Research in Reflexive Relationships. *Qualitative Inquiry*, 13, 5: 599–616.

Ettorre, E. (2005). Gender, Older Female Bodies and Autoethnography: Finding My Feminist Voice by Telling My Illness Story. *Women's Studies International Forum*, 28, 6: 535–546.

Eustachewich, L. (2017). *US Military Blows Millions a Year on Viagra for Its Troops*. Available at: https://nypost.com/2017/07/26/us-military-blows-millions-a-year-on-viagra-for-its-troops/ [Accessed: November 2, 2017].

Fairfield, M.A. (2004). Gestalt Groups Revisited: A Phenomenological Approach. *Gestalt Review*, 8, 3: 336–357.

Fallon, S. (2012). Sex, Gender, and the Theatre of Self: Acting Theory in (Gestalt) Psychotherapy with a Transsexual Client. *Gestalt Review*, 16, 2: 162–180.

Feder, B. and Ronall, R. (Eds.). (1980). *Beyond the Hot Seat: Gestalt Approaches to Group*. New York: Brunner/Mazel.

Finkelstein, P., Wenegrat, B. and Yalom, I. (1982). Large Group Awareness Training. *Annual Review of Psychology*, 33, 1: 515–539.

Finlay, L. (2011). *Phenomenology for Therapists: Researching the Lived World*: Chichester, Sussex: Wiley.

Finlay, L. and Evans, K. (2009). *Relational-centred Research for Psychotherapists: Exploring Meanings and Experience*. Chichester, Sussex: Wiley-Blackwell.

Fisher, J.D. (1990). *Evaluating a Large Group Awareness Training: A Longitudinal Study of Psychosocial Effects*. New York: Springer-Verlag.

Flansted-Jensen, E. (2008). Commentary IV: 'Gender Differences in Gestalt Therapy' – Doing Gender in Gestalt Therapy. *Gestalt Review*, 12, 2: 134–139.

Fogel, G.I. (2009). Interiority and Inner Genital Space in Men: What Else Can Be Lost in Castration? In: Reis, B. and Grossmark, R. (Eds.), *Heterosexual Masculinities: Contemporary Perspectives from Psychoanalytic Gender Theory*. New York: Taylor & Francis, pp. 231–260.

Forsyth, D.R. and Corazzini, J.G. (2000). Groups as Change Agents. In: Snyder, C.R. and Ingram, R.E. (Eds.), *Handbook of Psychological Change: Psychotherapy Processes and Practices for the 21st Century*. New York: Wiley, pp. 309–336.

Foucault, M. (1990). *The History of Sexuality: An Introduction*. New York: Random House Incorporated.

Foucault, M. (2003). *The Birth of the Clinic: An Archaeology of Medical Perception*. London: Routledge.

Foulkes, S.H. (1975). Problems of the Large Group from a Group-Analytic Point of View. In: Kreeger, L. (Ed.), *The Large Group: Dynamics and Therapy*. London: Karnac Books, pp. 33–56.

Fox, N.J. (2012). *The Body*. Cambridge: Polity.

Fox, N.J. and Alldred, P. (2017). *Sociology and the New Materialism: Theory, Research, Action*. Los Angeles: SAGE Publications.

Francesetti, G. (2015). From Individual Symptoms to Psychopathological Fields. Towards a Field Perspective on Clinical Human Suffering. *British Gestalt Journal*, 24, 1: 5–19.

Frank, R. (2001). *Body of Awareness: A Somatic and Developmental Approach to Psychotherapy*. Cambridge, MA: Gestalt Press.

Frank, R. and Barre, F.L. (2011). *The First Year and the Rest of Your Life: Movement, Development, and Psychotherapeutic Change*. New York: Taylor & Francis.

Frie, R. and Orange, D. (2013). *Beyond Postmodernism: New Dimensions in Clinical Theory and Practice*. Hove: Taylor & Francis.

Frolic, A. (2011). Who Are We When We Are Doing What We Are Doing? The Case for Mindful Embodiment in Ethics Case Consultation. *Bioethics*, 25, 7: 370–382.

Furneaux, H. (2014). Victorian Sexualities. *Discovering Literature: Romantics and Victorians*. Available at: www.bl.uk/romantics-and-victorians/articles/victorian-sexualities [Accessed: November 1, 2016].

Gabbard, G.O. (1996). *Love and Hate in the Analytic Setting*. Lanham, MD: Rowman & Littlefield Publishers.

Gadamer, H.-G. (2012). *Truth and Method*. New York: Continuum.

Gapp, K., Jawaid, A., Sarkies, P., Bohacek, J., Pelczar, P., Prados, J., Farinelli, L. Miska, E. and Mansuy, I.M. (2014). Implication of Sperm RNAs in Transgenerational Inheritance of the Effects of Early Trauma in Mice. *Natural Neuroscience*, 17, 5: 667–669.

Geertz, C. (2000). *Available Light: Anthropological Reflections on Philosophical Topics*. Princeton, NJ: Princeton University Press.

Gendlin, E.T. (2010). *Focusing*. London: Ebury Publishing.

Giuliano, F. (2011). Neurophysiology of Erection and Ejaculation. *Journal of Sexual Medicine*, 8: 310–315.

Goodman, P. (2010). *Drawing the Line Once Again: Paul Goodman's Anarchist Writings*. Oakland: PM Press.

Grant, A. (2010). Autoethnographic Ethics and Rewriting the Fragmented Self. *Journal of Psychiatric and Mental Health Nursing*, 17, 2: 111–116.

Grant, A. (2019). Dare to Be a Wolf: Embracing Autoethnography in Nurse Educational Research. *Nurse Education Today*, 82: 88–92. https://doi.org/10.1016/j.nedt. 2019.07.006.

Grant, A. and Zeeman, L. (2012). Whose Story Is It? An Autoethnography Concerning Narrative Identity. *Qualitative Report*, 17, 36, pp. 1–12.

Grant, A., Short, N.P. and Turner, L. (2013). Introduction: Storying Life and Lives. In: Short, N.P., Turner, L. and Grant, A. (Eds.), *Contemporary British Autoethnography*. Rotterdam: SensePublishers, pp. 1–16.

Gray, S.A.O., Jones, C.W., Theall, K.P., Glackin, E. and Drury, S.S. (2017). Thinking across Generations: Unique Contributions of Maternal Early Life and Prenatal Stress to Infant Physiology. *Journal of the American Academy of Child and Adolescent Psychiatry*, 56, 11: 922–929. https://doi.org/10.1016/j.jaac.2017.09.001.

Grossmark, R. (2009). Two Men Talking: The Emergence of Multiple Masculinities in Psychoanalytic Treatment. In: Reis, B. and Grossmark, R. (Eds.), *Heterosexual Masculinities: Contemporary Perspectives from Psychoanalytic Gender Theory*. New York: Taylor & Francis, pp. 73–88.

Grosz, E. (2010). Feminism, Materialism, and Freedom. In: Coole, D. and Frost, S. (Eds.), *New Materialisms: Ontology, Agency, and Politics*. Durham, NC: Duke University Press, pp. 139–157.

Gruppetta, M. (2004). Autophenomenography? Alternative Uses of Autographically Based Research. *AARE: Association for Active Researchers in Education Conference Paper Abstracts*. Available from: www.aare.edu.au/data/publications/2004/gru04228. pdf. Conference: Melbourne, 28 November – 2 December [Accessed: November 1, 2019].

Hajcak, F. and Garwood, P. (1987). *Hidden Bedroom Partners: Needs and Motives that Destroy Sexual Pleasure*. San Diego: Libra Publishers, Incorporated.

Harris, J.B. (1994). *Working with Large Groups and Teams*. Available from: www.mgc.org.uk/online-articles-2/ [Accessed: December 30, 2013].

Hawley, D.A. (2011). Therapeutic Work with Gender Identity Issues: A Response to John l. Bennett. *British Gestalt Journal*, 20, 1: 14–20.

Haywood, C. and Mac an Ghaill, M. (2003). *Men and Masculinities*. Buckingham: Open University Press.

Hearn, J. and Pringle, K. (2006). *European Perspectives on Men and Masculinities: National and Transnational Approaches*. Basingstoke, Hants: Palgrave Macmillan UK.

Herman, J.L. (2015). *Trauma and Recovery: The Aftermath of Violence – From Domestic Abuse to Political Terror*. New York: Basic Books.

Hodges, C. (2003). Creative Processes in Gestalt Group Therapy. In: Spagnuolo Lobb, M. and Amendt-Lyon, N. (Eds.), *Creative License: The Art of Gestalt Therapy*. Wien: Springer, pp. 249–260.

Holland, F. (1992). Aspects of Homosexuality. In: Siegel, E.V. (Ed.), *Psychoanalytic Perspectives on Women*. New York: Brunner/Mazel, pp. 89–99.

Husserl, E. (1960). *Cartesian Meditations: An Introduction to Phenomenology*. Hague: Springer.

Husserl, E. and Kersten, F. (1983). *Ideas Pertaining to a Pure Phenomenology and to a Phenomenological Philosophy: First Book: General Introduction to a Pure Phenomenology*. Hague: Springer.

Hycner, R.H. and Jacobs, L. (1995). *The Healing Relationship in Gestalt Therapy: A Dialogic – Self-Psychology Approach*. Gouldsboro: Gestalt Journal Press.

Hyde, C. (2006). Interpreting the Countertransference Erection: On Transformation and the Therapist's Internal Experience. *Smith College Studies in Social Work*, 76, 4: 67–77.

Iida, M., Shrout, P.E., Laurenceau, J. and Bolger, N. (2012). Using Diary Methods in Psychological Research. In: Cooper, H., (Ed.), *APA Handbook of Research Methods in Psychology: Foundations, Planning, Measures and Psychometrics, Vol. 1*. Washington DC: American Psychological Association, pp. 277–305.

Irvine, J.M. (2014). Is Sexuality Research 'Dirty Work'? Institutionalized Stigma in the Production of Sexual Knowledge. *Sexualities*, 17, 5–6: 632–656.

Island, T.K. (2003). The Large Group and Leadership Challenges in a Group Analytic Training Community. In: Schneider, S. and Weinberg, H. (Eds.), *The Large Group Revisited: The Herd, Primal Horde, Crowds and Masses*. London: Jessica Kingsley Publishers, pp. 201–2013.

Jacobs, L. (1996). Shame in the Therapeutic Dialogue. In: Wheeler, G. and Lee, R. (Eds.), *The Voice of Shame: Silence and Connection in Psychotherapy*. San Francisco: Jossey-Bass Publishers, pp. 297–314.

Jacobs, L. (2009). Relationality: Foundational Assumption. In: Ullman, D. and Wheeler, G. (Eds.), *Cocreating the Field: Intention and Practice in the Age of Complexity*. New York: Gestalt Press Book, pp. 41–66.

Jacobs, L. (2011). Critiquing Projection: Supporting Dialogue in a Post-Cartesian World. In: Bar-Yoseph Levine, T. (Ed.), *Gestalt Therapy: Advances in Theory and Practice*. Hove: Routledge, pp. 59–70.

Jacobs, L.M. (2017). Hopes, Fears, and Enduring Relational Themes. *British Gestalt Journal*, 26, 1: 7–16.

Jacobs, L.M. (2014). Learning to Love White Shame and Guilt: Skills for Working as a White Therapist in a Racially Divided Country. *International Journal of Psychoanalytic Self Psychology*, 9, 4: 297–312.

Johnson, R. (2014). Contacting Gender. *Gestalt Review*, 18, 3: 207–225.

Johnson, S.M. (1994). *Character Styles*. New York: W.W. Norton & Co Inc.

Jones, S.L.H., Adams, T.E. and Ellis, C. (2013). *Handbook of Autoethnography*. Walnut Creek, CA: Left Coast Press, Incorporated.

Joyce, P. and Sills, C. (2009). *Skills in Gestalt Counselling & Psychotherapy*. Los Angeles: SAGE Publications.

Karpman, S. (1968). Fairy Tales and Script Drama Analysis. *Transactional Analysis Bulletin*. Available at: www.karpmandramatriangle.com/pdf/DramaTriangle.pdf [Accessed: November 17, 2017].

Katz, D. and Kahn, R.L. (1966). *The Social Psychology of Organizations*. New York: Wiley.

Kaufman, G. (1980). *Shame: The Power of Caring*. Cambridge: Schenkman Publishing Company.

Kennedy, D.J. (2013). *Healing Perception: An Application of the Philosophy of Merleau-Ponty to the Theoretical Structures of Dialogic Psychotherapy*. Queensland, Australia: Ravenwood Press and Create Space Publishers.

Kepner, E. (2008). Gestalt Group Process. In: Feder, B. and Frew, J. (Eds.), *Beyond the Hot Seat Revisited: Gestalt Approaches to Group*. New Orleans, LA: The Gestalt Institute Press, pp. 17–38.

Kepner, J. (2008). Commentary II: Gender Differences in Gestalt Therapy. *Gestalt Review*, 12, 2: 124–130.

Kimmel, M.S. (2012). *The History of Men: Essays on the History of American and British Masculinities*. Albany: State University of New York Press.

Kincel, A. (2015a). Large Groups, Collective Gestalts and Prejudices: Autoethnographic Reflections of Attending Large Groups in Training. *British Gestalt Journal*, 24, 1: 45–53.

Koffka, K. (1935). *Principles of Gestalt Psychology*. New York: Harcourt.

Kohut, H. (1976). Creativeness, Charisma, Group Psychology. In: Ornstein, P. (Ed.), *The Search for the Self*. New York: International Universities Press, pp. 793–843.

Kolmannskog, V. (2014). Gestalt Approach to Gender Identity Issues: A Case Study of a Transgender Therapy Group in Oslo. *Gestalt Review*, 18, 3: 244–260.

Kreeger, L. (1975). *The Large Group: Dynamics and Therapy*. London: Karnac Books.

Law, J. (2004). *After Method: Mess in Social Science Research*. London: Taylor & Francis.

LeCompte, M.D. and Schensul, J.J. (2010). *Designing and Conducting Ethnographic Research*. Lanham: AltaMira Press.

Lee, R. (1995). Gestalt and Shame: The Foundation for a Clearer Understanding of Field Dynamics. *British Gestalt Journal*, 4, 1: 14–22.

Lee, R.G. (2007). Shame and Belonging in Childhood: The Interaction between Relationship and Neurobiological Development in the Early Years of Life. *British Gestalt Journal*, 16, 2: 57–83.

Levinas, E. (2012). *Totality and Infinity: An Essay on Exteriority*. Dordrecht: Kluwert Academic Publishers.

Levine, J.M. and Hogg, M. (Eds.). (2010). *Encyclopedia of Group Processes & Intergroup Relations*. Los Angeles: SAGE Publications.

Levine, P.A. (1997). *Waking the Tiger: Healing Trauma: The Innate Capacity to Transform Overwhelming Experiences*. Berkeley, CA: North Atlantic Books.

Lewin, K. (1952). *Field Theory in Social Science*. London: Tavistock Publications.

Loe, M. (2006). The Viagra Blues: Embracing or Resisting the Viagra Body. In: Rosenfeld, D. and Faircloth, C. (Eds.), *Medicalized Masculinities*. Philadelphia: Temple University Press, pp. 21–44.

Louis, É. (2019). *Who Killed My Father*. London: Vintage Publishing.

Lowen, A. (1994). *Bioenergetics*. London and New York: Penguin/Arkana.

Lukensmeyer, C. (2013). Creating Democratic Spaces: Citizen Engagement and Large Systems Change in Post-Katrina New Orleans. In: Melnick, J. and Nevis, E.C. (Eds.), *Mending the World: Social Healing Interventions by Gestalt Practitioners Worldwide*. Santa Cruz: Gestalt Press, pp. 92–111.

Mac an Ghaill, M. and Haywood, C. (2011). Schooling, Masculinity and Class Analysis: Towards an Aesthetic of Subjectivities. *British Journal of Sociology of Education*, 32, 5: 729–744.

Main, T. (1975). Some Psychodynamics of Large Groups. In: Kreeger, L. (Ed.), *The Large Group: Dynamics and Therapy*. London: Karnac Books, pp. 57–86.

Maltz, W. (2010). The Porn Trap. *Therapy Today*, 21, 1: 10–17.

Marivoet, D. (2017). Ethics and Embodiment. In: Prengel, S. (Ed.), *Somatic Perspectives on Psychotherapy*. Available at: https://somaticperspectives.com/marivoet-ethics-embodiment/ [Accessed: August 25, 2017].

McCormack, M. (2012). *The Declining Significance of Homophobia: How Teenage Boys Are Redefining Masculinity and Heterosexuality*. New York: Oxford University Press.

McElroy, D. (2013). Vladimir Putin Claims Russia is Moral Compass of the World. *The Telegraph*, 12 December 2013. Available at: www.telegraph.co.uk/news/worldnews/europe/russia/10513330/Vladimir-Putin-claims-Russia-is-moral-compass-of-the-world.html [Accessed: November 2, 2017].

Melnick, J. (2017). A Gestalt Approach to Social Change. *British Gestalt Journal*, 26, 1: 17–27.

Memorandum of Understanding on Conversion Therapy in the UK. (2015). *UK Council for Psychotherapy*. Available at: www.psychotherapy.org.uk/wp-content/uploads/2016/09/Memorandum-of-understanding-on-conversion-therapy.pdf [Accessed: June 20, 2016].

Merleau-Ponty, M. (2005). *Phenomenology of Perception*. London: Routledge Classics.

Merleau-Ponty, M. and Lefort, C. (1968). *The Visible and the Invisible: Followed by Working Notes*. Evanston: Northwestern University Press.

Metta, M. (2013). Putting the Body on the Line: Embodied Recovery Through Domestic Violence. In: Holman Jones, S.L., Adams, T.E. and Ellis, C. (Eds.), *Handbook of Autoethnography*. Walnut Creek, CA: Left Coast Press, Incorporated, pp. 486–510.

Miller, T. and Bell, L. (2012). Consenting to What? Issues of Access, Gate-Keeping and 'Informed' Consent. In: Miller, T., Birch, M., Mauthner, M. and Jessop, J. (Eds.), *Ethics in Qualitative Research*. Los Angeles: SAGE Publications, pp. 61–75.

Milska-Wrzosińska, Z. (2002). *Co wolno gejom?* Available at: www.archiwum.wyborcza.pl/Archiwum/1,0,1806863,20020802RPDGW,Co_wolno_Gejom,.html [Accessed: November 2, 2017].

Mindell, A. (1995). *Sitting in the Fire: Large Group Transformation Using Conflict and Diversity*. Portland, OR: Lao Tse Press.

Montorsi, F., Padma-Nathan, H. and Glina, S. (2006). Erectile Function and Assessments of Erection Hardness Correlate Positively with Measures of Emotional Well-Being, Sexual Satisfaction, and Treatment Satisfaction in Men with Erectile Dysfunction Treated with Sildenafil Citrate (Viagra). *Urology*, 68, 3A: 26–37.

Morgan, D. (2004). Class and Masculinity. In: Kimmel, M.S., Hearn, J. and Connell, R.W. (Eds.), *Handbook of Studies on Men and Masculinities*. Los Angeles: SAGE Publications, pp. 165–177.

Moustakas, C. (1990). *Heuristic Research*. Newbury Park, London, and New Delhi: SAGE.

Nevis, E.C. and Melnick, J. (2009). Gestalt Concepts as Applied to Social Change Intervention. In: Melnick, J. and Nevis, E.C. (Eds.), *Mending the World: Social Healing Interventions by Gestalt Practitioners Worldwide*. Santa Cruz: Gestalt Press, pp. 25–43.

NICE. (2019). *Antidepressant Drugs*. Available at: https://bnf.nice.org.uk/treatment-summary/antidepressant-drugs.html [Accessed: December 1, 2019].

Nichol, L. (2005). *The Essential David Bohm*. London: Routledge, Taylor & Francis.

Novack, J., Park, S.J. and Friedman, A.N. (2013). Integrated Masculinity: Using Gestalt Counseling with Male Clients. *Journal of Counseling and Development*, 91, 4: 387–507.

O'Neill, R.M., Constantino, M.J. and Mogle, J. (2012). Does Agazarian's Systems-centered® Functional Subgrouping Improve Mood, Learning and Goal Achievement? A Study in Large Groups. *Group Analysis*, 45, 3: 375–390.

O'Shea, L. (2000). Sexuality: Old Struggles and New Challenges. *Gestalt Review*, 4: 8–25.

O'Shea, L. (2016). Poetics of the Erotic. *British Gestalt Journal*, 25, 2: 66–70.

Ollendorff Reich, I. (1969). *Wilhelm Reich: A Personal Biography*. London: ELEK.

Orbach, S. (2010). *Bodies*. London: Profile Books.

Parlett, M. (1991). Reflections of Field Theory. *British Gestalt Journal*, 1, 2: 68–91.

Parlett, M. (2014). The Impact of War. *British Gestalt Journal*, 23, 1: 5–12.

Parlett, M. (2015). *Future Sense: Five Explorations of Whole Intelligence for a World that's Waking Up*. Kibworth Beauchamp: Troubador Publishing.

Perls, F. (1969). *Gestalt Therapy Verbatim*. Moab, UT: Real People Press.

Perls, F. (1978). *The Gestalt Approach & Eye Witness to Therapy*. New York: Bantam Books.

Perls, F. (2017). *Gestalt Therapy – Concepts and Approach of the Gestalt Therapy*. Available at: http://gestalttheory.com/quotes/ [Accessed: November 15, 2017].

Perls, F. and Wysong, J. (1992). *Ego, Hunger and Aggression: A Revision of Freud's Theory and Method*. Gouldsboro: Gestalt Journal Press.

Perls, F., Hefferline, R.F. and Goodman, P. (2003). *Gestalt Therapy: An Excitement and Growth in the Human Personality*. London: Souvenir Press.

Philippson, P. (2010). *Discussing at the Conference: Lost in Transformation? – Changing Identities in a Changing World*. Berlin: European Association for Gestalt Therapy.

Philippson, P. (2014a). Failure to Launch. *British Gestalt Journal*, 23, 1: 35–38.

Philippson, P. (2014b). Plenary Panel. Paper Read at *Exploring the Diversity of Gestalt Therapy*. Asilomar, California.

Pillow, W. (2003). Confession, Catharsis, or Cure? Rethinking the Uses of Reflexivity as Methodological Power in Qualitative Research. *International Journal of Qualitative Studies in Education*, 16, 2: 175–196.

Pines, M. (2003). Foreword. In: Schneider, S. and Weinberg, H. (Eds.), *The Large Group Re-visited: The Herd, Primal Horde, Crowds and Masses*. London: Jessica Kingsley Publishers, pp. 9–12.

Polster, E. (1995). *A Population of Selves: A Therapeutic Exploration of Personal Diversity*. Gouldsboro: The Gestalt Journal Press.

Polster, E. and Polster, M. (1973). *Gestalt Therapy Integrated: Contours of Theory and Practice*. New York: Brunner/Mazel.

Protevi, J. (2014). Body. In: Lawlor, L. and Nale, J. (Eds.), *The Cambridge Foucault Lexicon*. Cambridge: Cambridge University Press, pp. 51–56.

Ranke-Heinemann, U. (1994). *Putting Away Childish Things: The Virgin Birth, the Empty Tomb, and Other Fairy Tales You Don't Need to Believe to Have a Living Faith*. San Francisco: Harper.

Real, T. (1999). *I Don't Want to Talk About It: Overcoming the Secret Legacy of Male Depression*. New York: Scribner.

Reale, G. and Catan, J.R. (1990). *A History of Ancient Philosophy I: From the Origins to Socrates*. Albany: State University of New York Press.

Reich, W. and Carfagno, V. (1980). *Character Analysis*. New York: Farrar, Straus and Giroux.

Renn, P. (2013). Moments of Meeting: The Relational Challenges of Sexuality in the Consulting Room. *British Journal of Psychotherapy*, 29, 2: 135–153.

Renold, E. and Mellor, D. (2013). Deleuze and Guattari in the Nursery: Towards an Ethnographic Multi-Sensory Mapping of Gendered Bodies and Becomings. In: Coleman, R. and Ringrose, J. (Eds.), *Deleuze and Research Methodologies*. Edinburgh: Edinburgh University Press, pp. 23–41.

Resnick, R. (1997). The 'Recursive Loop' of Shame: An Alternate Gestalt Therapy Viewpoint. *Gestalt Review*, 1, 3: 256–269.

Richardson, L. (2000). Writing: A Method of Inquiry. In: Denzin, N.K. and Lincoln, Y.S. (Eds.), *The SAGE Handbook of Qualitative Research*. Thousand Oaks: SAGE Publications, pp. 923–948.

Robine, J.-M. (2007). Gestalt Therapy as Aesthetics. *International Gestalt Journal*, 30, 1: 9–30.

Robine, J.M. (2015). *Social Change Begins with Two*. Siracusa: Istituto di Gestalt HCC Italy.

Roccas, S. and Brewer, M.B. (2002). Social Identity Complexity. *Personality and Social Psychology Review*, 6, 2: 88–106.

Rodgers, A.B., Morgan, C.P., Leu, N.A. and Bale, T.L. (2015). Transgenerational Epigenetic Programming via Sperm Microrna Recapitulates Effects of Paternal Stress. *Proceedings of the National Academy of Sciences*, 112, 44: 13699–13704.

Romanyshyn, R.D. (2007). *The Wounded Researcher: Research with Soul in Mind*. New Orleans, LA: Spring Journal Books.

Rosenfeld, D. and Faircloth, C. (2006). *Medicalized Masculinities*. Philadelphia: Temple University Press.

Ruffolo, D.V. (2012). *Post-Queer Politics*. Farnham: Ashgate Publishing Limited.

Ruppert, F. (2008). *Trauma, Bonding & Family Constellations: Understanding and Healing Injuries of the Soul*. Frome: Green Balloon Publishing.

Rust, M.J. and Totton, N. (2012). *Vital Signs: Psychological Responses to Ecological Crisis*. London: Karnac Books.

Salih, S. (2002). *Judith Butler*. London: Routledge.

Salonia, G. (2016). *The Moon is Made of Cheese*. Ragusa, Rome, Venice: Gestalt Therapy Kairos Institute.

Samuels, A. (2003). From Sexual Misconduct to Social Justice. In: Mann, D. (Ed.), *Erotic Transference and Countertransference*. Hove: Taylor & Francis, pp. 138–56.

Samuels, A. (2016). *Men's Issues in Psychotherapy and Counselling*. Paper Read at Webinar by nscience UK, 12 March 2016.

Scheler, M. (2017). *The Nature of Sympathy*. Abingdon: Taylor & Francis.

Schneider, S. and Weinberg, H. (2003). *The Large Group Re-visited: The Herd, Primal Horde, Crowds and Masses*. London: Jessica Kingsley Publishers.

Seidler, V.J.J. (1997). *Man Enough: Embodying Masculinities*. London: SAGE Publications.

Sela-Smith, S. (2002). Heuristic Research: A Review and Critique of Moustakas's Method. *Journal of Humanistic Psychology*, 42: 52–88.

Shapiro, S.A. (1996). The Embodied Analyst in the Victorian Consulting Room. *Gender and Psychoanalysis*, 1, 3: 297–322.

Siegel, D.J. (2010). *Mindsight: The New Science of Personal Transformation*. New York: Bantam Press, Random House Publishing Group.

Simon, B. (2004). *Identity in Modern Society: A Social Psychological Perspective*. Oxford: Blackwell Publishing.

Simpson, J.A., Wilson, C.L. and Winterheld, H.A. (2004). Sociosexuality and Romantic Relationships. In: Harvey, J.H., Wenzel, A., Wenzel, C.A.P.A. and Sprecher, S. (Eds.), *The Handbook of Sexuality in Close Relationships*. Mahwah, NJ: Taylor & Francis, pp. 87–112.

Skaife, S.E. and Jones, K. (2008). The Art Therapy Large Group as a Teaching Method for the Institutional and Political Aspects of Professional Training. *Learning in Health and Social Care*, 8, 3: 200–209.

Skynner, A.C.R. (1975). The Large Group in Training. In: Kreeger, L. (Ed.), *The Large Group: Dynamics and Therapy*. London: Karnac Books, pp. 227–251.

Slavin, J.H., Oxenhandler, N., Seligman, S., Stein, R. and Davies, J.M. (2004). Dialogues on Sexuality in Development and Treatment. *Studies in Gender and Sexuality*, 5, 4: 371–418.

Sletvold, J. (2014). *The Embodied Analyst: From Freud and Reich to Relationality*. London: Taylor & Francis.

Solzhenitsyn, A.I. (1977). *Prussian Nights: A Narrative Poem*. Glasgow: Collins, Harvill Press.

Spagnuolo Lobb, M. (2009). Is Oedipus Still Necessary in the Therapeutic Room? Sexuality and Love Emerging at the Contact-boundary in a Situational Field. *Gestalt Review*, 13, 1: 47–61.

Sparkes, A. (2002a). Autoethnography: Self-Indulgence or Something More? In: Bochner, A.P. and Ellis, C. (Eds.), *Ethnographically Speaking: Autoethnography, Literature, and Aesthetics*. Walnut Creek, CA: AltaMira Press, pp. 209–232.

Sparkes, A. (2002b). *Telling Tales in Sport and Physical Activity: A Qualitative Journey*. Champaign, IL: Human Kinetics.

Sparkes, A. (2013). Autoethnography at the Will of the Body: Reflections on a Failure to Produce on Time. In: Short, N.P., Turner, L. and Grant, A. (Eds.), *Contemporary British Autoethnography*. Rotterdam: Sense Publisher, pp. 203–211.

Spinelli, E. (2005). *The Interpreted World: An Introduction to Phenomenological Psychology*. London: SAGE Publications.

Spraitz, J.D. and Bowen, K.N. (2016). Techniques of Neutralization and Persistent Sexual Abuse by Clergy: A Content Analysis of Priest Personnel Files from the Archdiocese of Milwaukee. *Journal of Interpersonal Violence*, 31, 15: 2515–2538.

Spry, T. (2001). Performing Autoethnography: An Embodied Methodological Praxis. *Qualitative Inquiry*, 7, 6: 706–732.

Spry, T. (2006). A 'Performative-I' Copresence: Embodying the Ethnographic Turn in Performance and the Performative Turn in Ethnography. *Text & Performance Quarterly*, 26, 4: 339–346.

Spry, T. (2011). *Body, Paper, Stage: Writing and Performing Autoethnography*. Walnut Creek, CA: Left Coast Press.

Staemmler, F.-M. (1997). On Cultivating Uncertainty: An Attitude for Gestalt Therapists. *British Gestalt Journal*, 6, 1: 40–48.

Staemmler, F.-M. (2010). Towards a Psychology of Joint Situation: From the Cult of Aggression to a Culture of Compassion. Paper Read at *Lost in Transformation?* European Association for Gestalt Therapy Conference, Berlin.

Staemmler, F.-M. (2012a). *Empathy in Psychotherapy: How Therapists and Clients Understand Each Other*. New York: Springer Publishing Company.

Staemmler, F.-M. (2012b). Self-Esteem, Compassion and Self-Compassion: From Individualism to Connectedness. *British Gestalt Journal*, 21, 2: 19–28.

Staemmler, F.-M. and Staemmler, B. (2009). Ego, Anger and Attachment: A Critique of Perls' Aggression Theory and Method. In: Staemmler, F.-M. (Ed.), *Aggression, Time, and Understanding: Contributions to the Evolution of Gestalt Therapy*. New York: The Gestalt Press, pp. 3–186.

Stanley, P. (2015). Writing the PhD Journey(s): An Autoethnography of Zine-Writing, Angst, Embodiment, and Backpacker Travels. *Journal of Contemporary Ethnography*, 44, 2: 143–168.

Stephan, C.W. and Bachman, G.F. (1999). What's Sex Got to Do With It? Attachment, Love Schemas, and Sexuality. *Personal Relationships*, 6, 1: 111–123.

Stern, D.N. (2000). *Interpersonal World of the Infant: A View from Psychoanalysis and Development Psychology*. New York: Basic Books.

Stets, J.E. (2006). Identity Theory. In: Burke, P.J. (Ed.), *Contemporary Social Psychological Theories*. Stanford: Stanford University Press, pp. 88–110.

Stevens, J.O. (2007). *Awareness*. Gouldsboro: The Gestalt Journal Press.

Stoller, P. (1997). *Sensuous Scholarship*. Philadelphia: University of Pennsylvania Press.

Swanson, J.L. (1982). The Paradox of the Safe Emergency. *The Gestalt Journal*, 5, 2: 57–64.

Tajfel, H. (1981). *Human Groups and Social Categories: Studies in Social Psychology*. Cambridge: Cambridge University Press.

Talmadge, L.D. and Talmadge, W.C. (1986). Relational Sexuality: An Understanding of Low Sexual Desire. *Journal of Sex & Marital Therapy*, 12, 1: 3–21.

Tamas, S. (2013). Who's There? A Week Subject. In: Jones, S.H., Adams, T.E. and Ellis, C. (Eds.), *Handbook of Autoethnography*. Walnut Creek, CA: Left Coast Press, Incorporated, pp. 186–202.

Taterka, A. (2017a). *Bioenergetic Gestalt Therapy in Practice: Pushing the Mattress*. [Drawing] (A. Kincel, private collection).

Taterka, A. (2017b). *Experimenting with Sexuality and Violation*. [Drawing] (A. Kincel, private collection).

Taterka, A. (2017c). *Fear of Homoeroticism in My Teenage Years: Andrew and Me*. [Drawing] (A. Kincel, private collection).

Taterka, A. (2017d). *Hot Seat Model as Modelled in My Training in Poland*. [Drawing] (A. Kincel, private collection).

Taterka, A. (2017e). *Large Group Session*. [Drawing] (A. Kincel, private collection).

Taterka, A. (2017f). *The Estate Where I Grew Up*. [Drawing] (A. Kincel, private collection).

Taterka, A. (2017g). *On the Knees of Tom: A Body Therapy and Heteronormativity*. [Drawing] (A. Kincel, private collection).

Taterka, A. (2017h). *Playing and Programming: 1988–1996*. [Drawing] (A. Kincel, private collection).

Taterka, A. (2017i). *Shaking Hands Experiment: Fear and Closeness*. [Drawing] (A. Kincel, private collection).

Taterka, A. (2017j). *Waiting for Admission to the 'Cool' Group*. [Drawing] (A. Kincel, private collection).

Taterka, A. (2017k). *An Advice from My Spelling Corrector*. [Drawing] (A. Kincel, private collection).

Taylor, G. (2005). *Integrating Quantitative and Qualitative Methods in Research*. Lanham: University Press of America, Incorporated.

Taylor, M.S. (2014). *Trauma Therapy and Clinical Practice: Neuroscience, Gestalt and the Body*. Maidenhead: Open University Press.

Terdiman, R. (2009). Given Memory: On Mnemonic Coercion, Reproduction and Invention. In: Radstone, S. and Hodgkin, K. (Eds.), *Memory Cultures: Memory, Subjectivity, and Recognition*. New Brunswick: Transaction Publishers, pp. 186–201.

Thomas, C. (2008). *Masculinity, Psychoanalysis, Straight Queer Theory: Essays on Abjection in Literature, Mass Culture, and Film*. Basingstoke: Palgrave Macmillan.

Todres, L. (2007). *Embodied Enquiry: Phenomenological Touchstones for Research, Psychotherapy and Spirituality*. Basingstoke: Palgrave Macmillan.

Tomasik, K. (2004). Co wolno psychologom? In: Sypniewski, Z. and Warkocki, B. (Eds.), *Homofobia po polsku*. Warszawa: Sic!.

Totton, N. (1998). *The Water in the Glass: Body and Mind in Psychoanalysis*. London: Rebus Press.

Tubbs, W. (1972). Beyond Perls. *Journal of Humanistic Psychology*, 12, 2: 77–79.

Turner, J.C. (1987). *Rediscovering the Social Group: A Self-Categorization Theory*. Oxford: Basil Blackwell.

Turquet, P. (1975). Threats to Identity in the Large Group. In: Kreeger, L. (Ed.), *The Large Group: Dynamics & Therapy*. London: Constable, pp. 87–144.

Twomey, D. (2003). British Psychoanalytic Attitudes towards Homosexuality. *Journal of Gay & Lesbian Psychotherapy*, 7, 1–2: 7–22.

United Kingdom Council for Psychotherapy (UKCP). (2009). *Ethical Principles and Code of Professional Conduct*. Available at: www.psychotherapy.org.uk/wp-content/uploads/2017/11/UKCP-Ethical-Principles-and-Code-of-Professional-Conduct.pdf [Accessed: December 7, 2017].

Vasseleu, C. (1998). *Textures of Light: Vision and Touch in Irigaray, Levinas and Merleau-Ponty*. London: Routledge.

Volkan, V.D. (2001). Transgenerational Transmissions and Chosen Traumas: An Aspect of Large-group Identity. *Group Analysis*, 34, 1: 79–97.

Warnecke, T. (2011). Stirring the Depths: Transference, Countertransference and Touch. *Body, Movement and Dance in Psychotherapy*, 6, 3: 233–243.

Wheeler, G. (1991). *Gestalt Reconsidered: A New Approach to Contact and Resistance*. New York: Gardner Press, Incorporated.

Wheeler, G. (1997). Self and Shame: A New Paradigm for Psychotherapy. In: Lee, R.G. and Wheeler, G. (Eds.), *The Voice of Shame: Silence and Connection in Psychotherapy*. Cambridge, MA: Gestalt Press, pp. 23–58.

Wheeler, G. (2006). New Directions in Gestalt Theory and Practice: Psychology and Psychotherapy in the Age of Complexity. *International Gestalt Journal*, 29, 1: 9–41.

Whitaker, D.S. (2001). *Using Groups to Help People*. Hove: Routledge.

Wikipedia. (2017). *National Association for Research & Therapy of Homosexuality*. Available at: https://en.wikipedia.org/wiki/National_Association_for_Research_%26_Therapy_of_Homosexuality [Accessed: December 1, 2017].

Willetts, M.C., Sprecher, S. and Beck, F.D. (2004). Overview of Sexual Practices and Attitudes within Relational Contexts. In: Harvey, J.H., Wenzel, A. and Sprecher, S. (Eds.), *The Handbook of Sexuality in Close Relationships*. Mahwah: Taylor & Francis, pp. 57–85.

Willig, C. (2008). *Introducing Qualitative Research in Psychology*. Maidenhead: McGraw-Hill Education.

Wollants, G. (2012). *Gestalt Therapy: Therapy of the Situation*. London: SAGE Publications.

Yehuda, R. and Bierer, L.M. (2009). The Relevance of Epigenetics to PTSD: Implications for the DSM-V. *Journal of Traumatic Stress*, 22, 5: 427–434.

Yehuda, R., Daskalakis, N.P., Bierer, L.M., Bader, H.N., Klengel, T., Holsboer, F. and Binder, E.B. (2016). Holocaust Exposure Induced Intergenerational Effects on FKBP5 Methylation. *Biological Psychiatry*, 80, 5: 372–380.

Yontef, G. (2009). The Relational Attitude in Gestalt Theory and Practice. In: Jacobs, L. and Hycner, R. (Eds.), *Relational Approaches in Gestalt Therapy*. New York: Routledge, Taylor & Francis Group, pp. 34–59.

Yontef, G. and Schulz, F. (2013). *Dialogic Relationship and Creative Techniques: Are They on the Same Team?* Los Angeles, CA: Pacific Gestalt Institute.

Yontef, G.M. (1993). *Awareness, Dialogue and Process: Essays on Gestalt Therapy*. Gouldsboro: The Gestalt Journal Press.

Zachary, A. (2001). Uneasy Triangles: A Brief Overview of the History of Homosexuality. *British Journal of Psychotherapy*, 17, 4: 489–492.

Zand, B. (2015). 'Culture War' of Gay Conversion Therapy. *BBC News*, 23 April 2015. Available at: www.bbc.com/news/uk-32397465 [Accessed: November 1, 2017].

Zeeman, L., Aranda, K. and Grant, A. (2014). Queer Challenges to Evidence-based Practice. *Nursing Inquiry*, 21, 2: 101–111.

Zeeman, L., Sherriff, N., Browne, K., McGlynn, N., Aujean, S., Pinto, N., Davis, R., Mirandola, M., Gios, L., Amaddeo, F., Donisi, V., Rosinska, M., Niedźwiedzka-Stadnik, M. and Pierson, A. (2017). *Comprehensive Scoping Report: A Review of the European Grey Literature on Health Inequalities Experienced by LGBTI People and the Barriers Faced by Health Professionals in Providing Healthcare for LGBTI People*. European Union: Health4LGBTI.

Zinker, J.C. (1977). *Creative Process in Gestalt Therapy*. New York: Brunner/Mazel.

Index

Page numbers in *italic* indicate a figure and page numbers in **bold** indicate a table on the corresponding page.

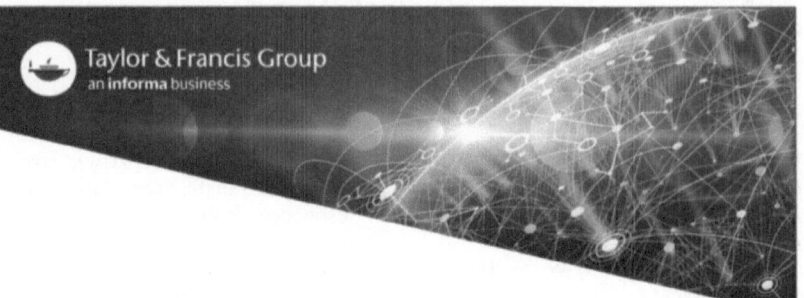
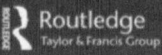
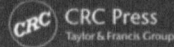